YOUR TOXIC WAIST

HEART ATTACKS, STROKES AND NOW. . . CANCER BUBBLE BELLY TROUBLE

Lawrence Power M. D.

CAUTION !

Obesity and heart disease, high blood pressure and diabetes are serious diseases that require professional supervision. This book is not a medical manual, although its intention is to help you to health yourself. Active patient participation is central to the best outcomes with today's major illnesses. Team up with your doctor. If you plan to lose weight, ask about all your medications. The ideal doctor-patient relationship is coach and player. Personal responsibility is not solo-care.

MEET DOCTOR POWER

Trained in Endocrinology and Metabolism at the University of Michigan, Dr. Power's academic credentials include professorships at the University of Michigan and at Wayne State University. His medical career has been spent in a variety of clinical settings in several countries around the world . . . in the active management, by rough count, of more than a hundred thousand patients. It was an experience that convinced him most people in the developed world suffer to a considerable extent from self-inflicted wounds. His years as Chief of Medicine at Detroit General Hospital had a huge influence on his thinking.

"Over a decade," he has written, as a national columnist with the Los Angeles Times Newspaper Syndicate, "the steady re-admission of discharged patients was a constant reminder of how short-lived were the successes of our best efforts. More durable outcomes would have resulted from teaching them strategies of self-care."

Dozens of individuals have contributed to this book . . . as teachers and colleagues. To all of them the author's debt is total, but his most important teachers have been those patients who provided the privilege of their confidence and insights.

Much research has tied food abundance and sedentary lifestyles to our killer diseases. Highlights have been collected for a free online game of baseball, divided into four skill levels: Grade 8, 12, undergraduate and graduate. Called HealthYourself101.com, it pitches the science bits, and here we connect the dots.

PROLOGUE

A Good Loser

My patient had a weight problem as well as high blood pressure, and was advised by an earlier physician to lose at least 30 pounds. But she'd been overweight for years, without high blood pressure, so they focused their attention on pills for the pressure. It kept the relationship harmonious, by focusing on blood pressure alone. Even in clinical settings, mentioning a patient's obesity carries a hint of rudeness. Nobody likes being fat.

She saw the doctor every three months and he judged the pressure to be well-controlled, although her weight continued to rise. Diabetes developed when she was 46. This time, after a week in hospital where she received dietary instruction—including the need to lose some weight. She'd been overweight for years, however, without diabetes or high blood pressure, so another pill was added to bring the sugar down, her weight politely ignored. More visits, more pills, more weight gain. It was not an unusual experience, indeed a typical history. She was 50 when she had the heart attack, and after discharge from hospital she experienced pain in her chest when exerting herself, the heart pain called angina. Still overweight, she underwent coronary artery bypass surgery.

    Throughout this medical odyssey, she had grown progressively large around the abdomen. It ran in the family, she would shrug, remarking that close relatives had lived into their nineties. What runs in families, however, are tendencies more often than diseases themselves. The tendency to be overweight is a genetic predisposition that expresses itself in the presence of abundance: an abundance of food, and an abundance of ease. Her bypass surgery was disappointing. It failed to relieve her breathlessness or fatigue, and she finally faced the problem of her weight by changing doctors. Over the next six months, she shed 43 excess pounds and was transformed. The diabetes disappeared. The high blood pressure disappeared. She no longer needed medication and was no longer tired or breathless. She was cured, or more correctly, came under biological control by taking responsibility for her health, specifically her toxic waist.

Now off all medication, she walks briskly for an hour every day and watches the flood of food enticements on television and through the mail, with a jaundiced eye. Her health insurance company paid out tens of thousands of dollars for her medical care - she once laughed, during an office visit - but refused to reimburse for the costs of the coaching she needed to control her weight . . . dollars for treatments, regrets for cure. It is not called the Health Care *Industry* by accident.

CONTENTS

TOTAL CALORIES DELIVERED INTO
THE US FOOD SUPPLY PER PERSON PER DAY

1970 2200 calories

1980 2200 calories

1990 2400 calories

2000 2500 calories

2010 2700 calories

SERIOUS HEALTH CARE

INVOLVES SKEPTICISM
REGARDING UTOPIAN MEDICINE,
A PREFERENCE FOR PERSONAL RESPONSIBILITY
AND HABIT CHANGE OVER HIGH TECHNOLOGY.

IT'S ABOUT KNOWLEDGEABLE SELF-CARE.

INTRODUCTION

A FEW PRELIMINARIES
READY HELPING HANDS:

Doctors,

Clinics,

Malls,

Mails.

Once upon a time the word diet meant your daily food intake. Today it means weight-loss and a food plan to make fat disappear. It will eventually mean portion control and daily exercise. Going hungry is not a natural circumstance but a necessary period of recovery from an environment of excess. Reduced portion size is a preparation for the next stage which is lifelong. Both can involve high tech help and real food. The purpose of portion control, using your fist size as your measurement, is to shrink your stomach, as is done surgically these days. Feeling in the know gets you out of victimhood by slowly introducing new food and fitness changes into your daily routine. Rely on clothing fit for your ongoing assessment, or ring size, at ease internally, with an absence of discomfort, not craving, not anxious, not itching, not restless. This book is mostly about the helping hand coming out of your own sleeve, but first a review of developments along lines currently available.

DOCTORS AND BARIATRIC CLINICS . . . The New Wave

Usually staffed by a physician, they often include teams of capable individuals skilled at food or fitness or psychology or motivation. Get to one if your weight problem is complicated by smoking or pregnancy or self-induced vomiting.

In the middle of the past century (1950-60) thyroid hormone was the treatment of choice for obesity, and complaints of fatigue or sensitivity to cold. The thyroid gland secretes two hormones, both thyroid, which help maintain body temperature, weight, muscle strength and fluid balance. As better tests of thyroid function became available they failed to reveal any under-activity of the thyroid gland for most patients being overweight. Doctors stopped calling the condition hypothyroidism although many continued to use thyroid for what they called a patient's 'hypo-metabolism'.

The problem with taking thyroid in such circumstances is that many are sensitive to its effects as a stimulant, developing increased heart rates, skipped beats and potentially fatal rhythm disorders. Other drugs were developed that found favor for a few years but were eventually abandoned because of complications like addiction or psychotic breaks..

Some physicians argue that drugs be used long-term in the management of obesity, like drugs for diabetes and hypertension that provide benefits day-to-day but are lost once the drug is stopped. Recently (in 2012) and for the first time in more than a decade, Food and Drug Administration officials approved two new weight-loss drugs. They are not for people who just want to drop a few pounds, but for those with 50 surplus pounds and some weight-related complication, such as hypertension, cholesterol, diabetes or sleep apnea. Your doctor may prescribe both, which brings up the possibility that drug support might soon become a useful adjunct to habit change regarding exercise and food portion control.

Safe and effective drugs are desperately needed in the struggle to cope with a rising tide of patients seeking surgery for their obesity or needing help with eating disorders. Look into these new developments. If you're struggling with a weight problem, you know it's the little things that add up . . . a little more at the buffet, a little more sitting around, a little snugness of the waist.

Giving up smoking commonly leads to weight gain. Some consider the cigarette a food substitute and smoke when they are hungry. Nicotine does decrease the appetite and is probably its greatest reason that smokers remain lean. It is even more destructive of your health than the toxic waist, so stopping must be given priority. Many smokers have reached a stage in the struggle to quit where they would benefit from a short-term appetite suppressant. What is needed is a safe suppressant that is non-addicting and mood-neutral. Clever chemists are hard at work on this problem world-wide.

Being pregnant and overweight poses a double jeopardy. Excessive weight can be associated with a condition called toxemia of pregnancy, but too little weight gain during pregnancy can harm the baby. Get proper supervision from a qualified physician/obstetrician during pregnancy, and do not go on any self-imposed diet.

Anorexia nervosa is an eating disorder typically met in younger women, who avoid food to the point of starvation. A few starve themselves to death. Usually bright and alert, they refuse to believe they are too thin, and may need hospital care.

Bulimia is an eating disorder characterized by recurring episodes of over-eating then purging through self-induced vomiting or the use of laxatives. It is a variant on anorexia and more common but not harmless. Both are expressions of the same forces . . . a society that encourages us as consumers to overeat, while admiring fashion models who are too thin.

Gastro-esophageal reflux disease (GERD) is rarely recognized as a weight-induced disorder, but a deficiency of antacids (in all the television tales). Weight loss decreases pressure on the stomach so stomach acid no longer seeps up where it burns.

BARIATRIC SURGERY

Among the surgical procedures developed by practitioners of this growing specialty, the stomach has been stapled, cut down in size, filled with a plastic balloon, and banded. Changing its size is based on the assumption that appetite is controlled by stomach distention which is only partly true.

Another approach involves attacking an innocent small intestine: bypassing food around a third of its digestive surface for controlled malabsorption. Complications from this desperate measure include diarrhea with fluid loss, liver failure, kidney failure, malnutrition and bone disease. Such patients require dedicated long-term management.

Liposuction directly attacks fat deposits, and consists of inserting a specialized suction tube through small incisions then forcing fat into the instrument's holes and tiny blade edges. The procedure works best to reduce unsightly bulges after weight loss from calorie restriction. In experienced hands the benefits are significant and the technique is undergoing steady improvement. For male patients it can help reduce breast bulges and abdominal 'handles'.

MALLS

Ubiquitous, commercial weight loss businesses provide a support network for overweight individuals. By encouraging fitness routines with regular supervision they do good work. Among a population of 50 participants who had lost at least 25 pounds in one commercial weight-loss operation, most had: more energy, less fatigue, less trouble breathing and sleeping, less acid indigestion, and no more aches or pains in their joints and limbs. Yet *before* losing weight: none had admitted to: feeling tired or lacking energy, having trouble with breathing or sleeping, having acid indigestion, having mild joint aches or pains.

By helping individuals lose 20-30 pounds, commercial weight-loss operations provide useful support systems, conventional advice and the support of monitoring. All of them publicize their short-term successes, but none provide five-year 'cure rates'. Hmmm. Once down to maintenance, the most enduring helping hands for you will be found coming out of your own sleeves. Develop a support network of new friends who are similarly into wellness, and who have taken personal responsibility for their health. Continue to enjoy the company of old friends around food by simply sipping some tea or coffee. A walking routine will eventually collect associates from the neighborhood, the workplace or your workout place: other wellness wonks looking for company.

Meals-by-mail is a means of portion control leaving too many problems hanging.

CONNECTING THE DOTS . . .
TO A HIGH BLOOD PRESSURE

EVEN THE SMALLEST BUBBLE BELLY . . .

. . . floods the liver with fatty acids,

. . . that slowly choke important machinery in liver cells,

. . . and allow excessive insulin into the circulation,

. . . which retains salt and plumps up the blood volume,

. . . that causes the blood pressure to rise,

. . . chunking cholesterol into artery walls to clutter them.

LOOKING FOR THE ACTION?
START HERE:

CHAPTER 1

YOUR OWN HELPING HANDS: CLEARING THE DECKS

Step 1

Because most readers will be approaching this book from the Batter's Box of HealthYourself101.com the usual arrangement of chapters has been set on its head. Up front and center you will find the FIVE STEPS my Prologue Patient took to be rid of her toxic waist. For a deeper depth of understanding of how we got into our national (and now global) predicament, with its lethal clinical extensions, ten chapters follow in logical progression. For now, let's lose some weight.

STEP ONE

1

Changing weighs is a bungee jump. More important than your weight next month or for the upcoming class reunion, is your weight next year, although some earlier return on the effort is gratifying. Double digit losses in the first week or two come from stored water and sugar. Called glycogen, large amounts of it in liver and muscle are used when calorie intakes fall. The released water is passed as urine and your weight falls. Only then will you begin burning fat. You will be eating about 800 calories a day of a low-fat, high protein intake that should be combined with a walking program.

First, a precaution: being overweight or hypertensive, diabetic or hypercholesterolemic are not risk-free states of health. Nor is correcting them a risk-free undertaking. Begin to change your ways prudently with the support and guidance of your health care provider.

Cigarette smokers and very overweight individuals are at increased risk of sudden death from any unaccustomed physical activity. Pain is a danger signal. If it occurs during exercise cut back or rest at the first sign. Pain tells you that too much is being asked, that fibers are being stretched or torn or that a demand for oxygen is not being met. Weakness has surfaced in the system, and you must stop hurting yourself. Fitness is a recreation. Only gradually should you push your limits back.

Get medical advice . . .

If you smoke

　　If your heart starts jumping or racing

If discomfort or pressure occurs in your chest or arms

If you experience dizziness or tend to black out

If you feel unusually tired after a workout

If you become severely short of breath

A supervised program, among the many that are commercially available, will enable you to enter the weight control big leagues. Going on and off a series of 'tabloid diets' produces nothing but exasperation. Tell your friends you're on a 'program' not a diet. Permanent control means disengaging yourself from our free-market food vendors.

Fats and oils deliver 42% of our daily calories, and are tightly associated with obesity, heart disease and cancer. Excessive salt is related to high blood pressure, while excessive refinement (a loss of fiber) robs food of appetite satisfaction, and helps promote obesity, diabetes, diverticulitis and bowel cancer.

In the interest of feeling better, looking better and having the energy of improved health we must return to an older, less glittering but more peace-able foodstyle. It is the food on which humankind evolved and one to which the human digestive tract accommodates quickly and quietly. It is a tranquil and relaxing foodstyle, an appetite-satisfying and disease-preventing one. Its preparation calls for a minimum of fuss and stress. It's mainstays are quick to fix. Take advantage of the convenience of technology like the freezer, the blender and the microwave oven. There's lots of nutritious, delicious stuff in the supermarkets. Go for them selectively. Be eccentric, and have some good clean fun.

Do not try to lose weight on your own if you take any prescription medicine or see a physician for any chronic disease. Weight loss inevitably means starvation (a controlled, intentionally low calorie intake). It means your body must begin burning some of the stored fat and inevitably tissue protein in large amounts. It means that the brain will be affected, the kidneys and liver and the muscles (the heart is a muscle). It means that you should not lose weight if you are pregnant or nursing. Sharing the guidance you find in this book with your personal physician is a prudent move. It is also a prudent practice to take a daily multivitamin when losing weight.

Clear out the cupboards and your refrigerator of all food off program if you live alone. Give them away to a food bank or homeless shelter. Because sugar and salt are hard-wired natural cravings, they will never go away. Rid your kitchen, your desk and your car of all sweets and salty or packaged snacks. If you live with others who also use the kitchen, set aside sections that are exclusively yours. Begin a regular walking saunter out of the office or from a house. You will soon find someone else who wants to join in.

The high-tech part of the program involves a protein powder commercially available in several flavors that helps suppress the appetite. Using the powder alone must only be done under weekly medical supervision. Certain blood minerals can get dangerously deranged, especially the serum potassium. For this reason an unsupervised program encourages no more than three protein drinks a day (1 scoop in a measure of fat-free or skim milk) ideally with berries such as raspberries, blueberries or chunked strawberries.

Three Simply Effective FITNESS Activities:

Walking:

Human beings have been walking upright for more than a million years. It is a simple activity once the basics are mastered, and requires no special equipment. The learning was done during your first two years of life. It is safe and available year round. It tones up the muscles, heart and lungs. It is a natural tranquilizer. It can be very sociable.

Dancing:

For many people dancing is a pleasant alternative to walking or jogging. And they are right. Many women – exhausted by the prospect of a 10 minute walk – could dance for hours, given agreeable music and company. It is an excellent combination of fitness and recreation, as are skating, skipping rope and rebounding.

Jogging:

There is no shortage of horror stories for anyone thinking about running: the overweight fellow found dead along the road or the middle-age heart attack victim who quits smoking, loses weight, starts to jog and has a second heart attack. Jogging is graduate level walking. Don't begin with it, and when you do begin, start slow and taper.

Each foot strikes the ground 1000 times during a mile of walking. Feet take a pounding over any distance, but even the fanciest of good footwear costs less than a dime a mile. A good walking or jogging shoe is cushioned to help absorb road shock (up to a third of the shock) thanks to layers of cushion. Wear comfortable athletic socks too.

Good shoes have a supporting plastic cup built-in around the heel. It's called the counter, and provides lateral stability, reducing heel wobble at the moment of contact. Excessive wobble leads to aching knees and ankles. The body's weight is normally distributed along the outer edge of the sole of the foot. The natural arch of a normal foot assures this distribution of weight and good shoes promote it with arch cushions built under the insole. There should be a soft role of binding around the mouth of the shoe and a tab rise over the heel. These protect the skin around the ankle and the Achilles' tendon.

Walking and running are simple, natural, sweaty, activities that can induce a childlike exuberance from the world of helpful technology on your feet. A dozen brands are competing for your trade with designer colors and fiercely tricky minor marketing points. If the shoe that catches your fancy has the support and features mentioned, try it on. If it fits and feels good buy it . One or two smart items of outerwear make sense as well, and some attractive wet wear. They make a statement about your commitment.

A Few Words About The 'Water Fast'

Water Fasting takes 2 weeks for any measurable body benefits, and ideally 3 or 4 weeks, done under medical supervision. It provides an opportunity to read and reflect, go for walks, put your house in order, write letters, update a journal, contact old friends, listen to music, meditate, enjoy walks around the neighborhood, or some hobby.

Many normal-weight people find fasting for short periods of time, an ideal mind-body restorative. Those who have discovered its benefits are not flagellants, nor foodists, nor are they holy men with hair shirts living on the edge of civilization.

A water fast provides a sharp reduction of calories for a defined period of time, often no longer than a week or week-end. Fluids are encouraged in the form of water and fruit or vegetable juices. Urine production in quantity facilitates a 'detoxification' effect.

Spiritual individuals, meditators and visualizers have taken advantage of the slight narcotic effect of fasting ketones on the brain to experience some transcendentalization. Ketone bodies are the smoke of burning fat. They can effect brain function in a mildly intoxicating way. It is a natural 'high' that takes several days to get into, but actually slows down higher brain skills like math and recall. Be careful while driving the car.

From Patients Who Practice Intermittent Fasting:

"It really clears the head by the second week. I understand its religious associations,"

"No more blood pressure pills. It restored my energy.'"
"It's my money-saving, spa alternative."
"It's nice not being tired all the time."
"There's a rewarding mental effect"

REGULAR VIGOROUS PHYSICAL ACTIVITY
PROMOTES A SENSE OF WELL-BEING,
AND IMPROVES PERFORMANCE OF ALL
BODY PARTS.

CHAPTER 2

YOUR OWN HELPING HANDS: TAKING THE PLUNGE

STEP 1

STEP 2

This is not a vegetarian program but vegetarians do live long and energetic lives. Lean meat, chicken and fish slivers can be part of your eventual diet. Think Asian. Cheese is loaded with cholesterol and saturated fat so use it sparingly, and for flavor: hard cheese grated over soups, into an egg-white mushroom omelet or crumbled into salads.

You Will Be Eating Six Times A Day,

AND A SERVING SIZE EACH TIME: THE SIZE OF YOUR CLENCHED FIST.

MAKE A FIST AND SEE HOW NICELY IT WOULD FIT INTO A RICE BOWL. THAT IS THE SIZE YOUR ELASTIC STOMACH WILL SHRINK DOWN TO ON ITS OWN, A SIZE YOU WILL SOON LEARN, FEELS BOTH SATISFIED AND FILLING. TWO FISTS ARE FOR SPECIAL, RARE CELEBRATIONS.

On an effective program you will lose 5-10 pounds the first week, living off stored sugar. It is stored in the muscles and liver and other tissues as a crystal called glycogen, which holds much water. Once the sugar is extracted and burned, the surplus water leaves the body creating great weight loss. Then tissue metabolism turns to fat. A pound a week thereafter is a reasonable and productive result. It is a program of portion control for life, a program and not a diet. Sadly, you must begin to look with a skeptical eye on the the mischievous charms of the free market and its blandishments to sit and eat. A sensible program works with your body as it exists, and as you know it. It provides nutritional choices that are simple and support full function while promoting a long life.

Dinner parties need all the planning you can muster. Explaining that you are on a program will only make them roll their eyes and isolate you socially. Tell no one that you are losing/controlling your weight. Eat before you go and spend dinner time cutting and shifting food around on your plate, all the while keeping a plate of salad at hand to feed from. Chat up your neighbors while sipping water and being a good guest.

Alcohol is important to some individuals whether as a social drink, a business drink, or while relaxing at home. Have no more than one a day, and seconds only for special occasions. Alcohol is a calorie source and common reason for program digression.

Your Six Eating Times Over The Day:

BREAKFAST MID-MORNING LUNCH
MID-AFTERNOON SUPPER EVENING

Your Food Options At Those Times:

PROTEIN POWDER SKIM MILK SHAKES (LIMIT 3 A DAY)
VEGETABLE SOUPS VEGETABLE SALADS
OAT & HONEY GRANOLA BARS EGG WHITE MUSHROOM
OMLETS
MICROWAVED VEGETABLES FRESH FRUITS & BERRIES

Some Daily Dietary Enhancements:

WATER, COFFEE, TEAS,
SPICES, LEMON JUICE, NONFAT DRESSING

A Few Suggested Additions:

BERRIES AND CREME (THICKEN UP A VANILLA PROTEIN
SCOOP)
GREEN BEANS AND SLIVERED TOASTED ALMONDS
A SCOOP OF BRAN IN A VANILLA PROTEIN DRINK
FOR NIGHT-TIME HUNGRIES: A PROTEIN SHAKE

Water Is A Convenient Stomach-Filler
At 6-8 Glasses A DAY

The best thirst quencher is plain tap water which all municipalities check regularly for purity. Use coffee or tea as your social food encounter edible when sitting down for a break with friends. Artificially sweetened drinks like diet sodas just keep a natural sweet craving alive. Avoid fruit juice for the same reason but eat fruit.

Any meal the size of your two bunched fists should make you feel 'stuffed'. That is the tailored size of your normal full stomach. A serving the size of one fist is for weight loss **and** weight control. The stomach is an elastic organ. It eventually shrinks down to where you will fill it with a single fist of food . . . reducing your stomach size without surgery. Hunger is an uncomfortable early feeling that will soon become low-grade and tolerable. It is the feeling of thin. Remind yourself that fat is being burned away.

Cravings tend to decrease as fat is burned. Ketone bodies do this. They are smoke from burning fat. They can have a barbiturate-like effect on the brain, sometimes producing a feeling of exuberant energy. As they rise in the blood they help suppress the appetite. Exercise pours ketone bodies into the blood. They are the reason that a brisk walk reduces cravings. Try a brisk walk instead of a snack and you will likely find the hunger gone. Take charge of your body. It looks to you for leadership.

Begin Taking Daily Breaks:

Daily walks are as crucial as calorie control for permanent weight loss. Numerous studies on many volunteers confirm this. Exercise equipment and machines are fine but walking is a basic human activity that requires nothing special except the decision to break your weight-gain routine. If you are into your middle years do not consider attacking a weight problem without first checking your cardiovascular system, lungs and legs. Get a thorough examination from a physician in whom you have confidence. Trips away from home or work and those inevitable 'special occasions' can be accommodated with granola bars, apples, oranges and bottled shakes. Take part in group celebrations with a cup of coffee or tea.

Exercise anytime that your schedule allows, remembering that . . .

Morning breaks burn more fat than evening breaks.

A fasting break burns more fat than a walk after any meal.

Cold weather burns more fat than exercise indoors or in summer.

Fat burning is not immediate, so aim for 30 minute breaks.

The trim unit of fitness: A mile in 15 minutes. Once achieved, take on 2 miles in 30 minutes, 3 miles in 45 and 4 in an hour. Done 5 - 6 times a week usually assures a lean body. Television and computers are today's great thieves of time and fitness.

It is a prudent practice to avoid sweets and salty snacks, while you develop a flavor preference for crisp and savory. Find like-minded colleagues or friends, or join a commercial weight-loss group. Your future should be oriented to real food, whole foods, fruits and vegetables. Keep your dishes simple. Use simple spices for greater flavor: mustard, oregano, curry powder, cumin or tarragon and basil. Use sprinkle cheese or tomato sauce. A drop of oil or a pinch of sugar is the most you should add to your food on the plate. Do not spend much time planning meals or thinking about food. Busy yourself with other interests.

Common Early Weight Loss Issues:

Feeling High: Burning body fat produces chemicals called ketones. Like alcohol, they lift the mood but you are not as sharp as you think. Be careful while driving your car. Be very wary of alcohol while losing weight.

Feeling shivery: You may feel chilly as your body hunkers down. Put on an extra sweater. It is not a sign of thyroid trouble.

Lightheadedness: You may feel that you are about to faint, especially when getting up from lying prone. It results from a shrinking blood volume. Change positions (getting up from a chair or out of bed) slowly. It is aggravated by hot weather, by sauna baths and by hot baths. Stay out of the heat and avoid hot tubs while losing weight. A cup of bouillon often takes care of such symptoms within an hour or so.

Dry Skin and Loose Hair: Rely on lotions for skin care. A slight itching rash during the first few days will respond to Calamine and disappears within a week. Hair growth stops during weight loss but returns with isocaloric eating. Scalp hair will come loose more readily while losing weight so do not have it "permed" or teased or dyed, nor brush it vigorously.

Strong Breath: can be managed by sucking breath sweeteners.

Easy Bruising: the result of a loss of cushioning fat and support structures around the tiniest blood vessels under the skin and their sheering with the slightest of bumps.

Cold Intolerance: from a loss of insulating fat particularly in cold weather.

Constipation: bran or a whole foods diet and water will usually solve it.

Depression: most hungry people are not happy about being hungry although a few become psychiatrically depressed and need medical help.

Diarrhea: sometimes occurs in response to too many salads or an intolerance of the high protein formula.

In summary, going without food commonly prompts feelings of fatigue, depression, difficulty in concentrating, and a sense of light-headedness when getting up too quickly from the sitting or recumbent position. Other complaints include: intestinal gas and constipation, and rarely gallbladder attacks or the painful arthritis of gout can complicate programs.

No Loss After A Week? Reduce Your Serving Sizes.

We human beings are omnivores, that is to say we need a variety of different foods in our diet for total nutrition. Other creatures do not, and happily thrive on chronic intakes of grass, insects or seeds. They "crave" nothing more, look for no flavor enhancers, no fresh variety. We are different. Mother Nature assures our dietary variety by driving us to seek it, by boring us when we eat the same food. We become turned off by the 'same old thing.' It is the flavors of today that fatten us.

Cravings can be mild or severe and excessive. Sometimes they are a displacing behavior, a substitute for some other activity denied. The tail-tapped rat tries to get away from the annoying tapping, and if escape is prevented, the rat will try to attack the tapper. If that is prevented it will turn to eating food or lapping water, whatever is available. The hazard of choosing fatty foods (e.g. ice cream) to satisfy a craving is a weight problem.

More calories are eaten during a meal consisting of several foods than during a meal of just one food, even if that food is a favorite. The more dissimilar the foods, the greater the intake. In a calorie-abundant culture such as ours, variety promotes obesity. After a Thanksgiving turkey dinner, who wants turkey for dessert? There's no room, but pumpkin pie? Yes, please. Variety defeats satiety.

CHAPTER 3

YOUR OWN HELPING HANDS:
THE EARLY WEEKS

STEP 1

STEP 2

STEP 3

Although more calories are burned when exercising in the cool out-of-doors, not all neighborhoods are safe, and the darker early hours of the cold months pose risks in the most public of open and lit parks. A piece of home exercise equipment – many effective ones are on the market – would make a sensible investment. Look first at those that keep you working out while on your feet, rather than your seat.

Those paragons of the work ethic – the bee, the ant and the beaver – only labor purposefully for about a third of their day. Another third of the time they rest, and the final third they appear to spend knocking about the neighborhood. The human equivalent would be going for a stroll: an important escape from the pressures of chores every day and a strategy to get unwound. When you can't leave your task or desk, have a mental device (like a soft word you can repeat to yourself in a rhythmic and hypnotic way) to produce a relaxed body.

The day's chores inevitably focus your mental energy on pre-occupying concerns, and tension builds in the muscles after an hour or so. Recharging is required, other than with chocolate or a cookie. If possible put your feet up. Let it all go for a minute or two. You are scratching an itch and it should feel good. Full health is a process that balances the day's activities so that needs, wants and obligations are regularly re-aligned. Studies have shown that we function best on a 12-hour cycle, starting at 6 in the morning and ending at 6 in the evening. We are most in synchrony with our tissues if we follow the rhythm of the sun, nature's basic time-giver for most of the body's clocks, and there are hundreds of them. When ignored, as in today's 24/7 lifestyle, dysrhythms result that reflect themselves in mood and performance. Too often, we scratch the itch with food.

We are muscled to rely on our hind legs, and need a variety of balancing reflexes and muscles to stay upright. The greatest return on human effort comes from exercise undertaken on our two feet . . . walking, dancing, jogging, running, skipping rope or rebounding. Machines that enable you to sit down or float or lie back do not provide the benefit of a comparable time at the effort. Use machines that work your walk.

Performance guide to Walking/Dancing

Take several weeks
    to get from 10 minutes a day to 30 minutes each day
Take several weeks more
    to get from a mile in 20 minutes to 2 in 30 minutes
Take more weeks
    to go from 3 miles an hour to 4 miles, 5 times a week

By then
you should be able to manage a Power Walk of 5 miles an hour.

Serpents in the Garden of Fitness

Simple overuse is the most common complication of any new fitness activity, and is to be expected. Complaints from body parts are the rule and not the exception. They are a signal to rest, cut back, heal up and regain the pace again. For problems that persist, that do not respond over time to rest and heat, see your doctor or a fitness expert.

Muscle soreness: usually results from tiny muscle fiber tears. Rest and a cold compresses the first day. Rest and heat on subsequent days.

Muscle cramps: an overused muscle contracts and stays contracted in a knot that you may feel. Rest it, massage it and gently stretch it. Cut back. Start over.

Muscle strain: usually results when a larger muscle fiber tears. Rest and cold for the first day. Rest and heat over subsequent days.

Side stitch: thought to be due to spasm of a segment of the diaphragm. Slowdown. Stop. Rest.

Tendon/ligament sprain: torn fibrous tissue around a joint where a muscle inserts. Rest and cold first day. Rest and heat on subsequent days. Tendons and ligaments do not have the circulation that muscles do. They take longer to heal.

Shin splints: a catchall term for tenderness in the front of the leg. Usually the result of minor muscle tears, but sometimes a stress fracture of the shin bone. Rest and cold first day. Rest and heat subsequent days but it's not improving within a few days, get help and perhaps an x-ray.

Calf pain: usually a result of overuse. In older individuals it may be a sign of diminished circulation. Cut back, rest and heal. If it recurrs at a certain level of activity get advice from a professional. It could mean narrowed arteries in the leg.

Heel pain: usually a bruised point or torn attachment. Not a "heel spur". The spur is not a spur at all, but a fleck of calcium in an old blood clot from long ago. It is not responsible for the pain which arises in fresh tendon and ligament tears around the area. Take pressure off the tender area by finding the tenderest spot and dabbing it with a felt-tipped pen. Place the inked bare foot into your walking shoe with a foam insole in place. Cut out the stained patch and reinsert the insole.

Arch pain: usually the result of torn plantar ligaments over the sole of the foot. Rest and cold compresses the first day. Rest and heat over subsequent days. Consider an arch support over the counter or having a professional prosthetic insert made to fit.

Achilles tendonitis: tenderness along the major heel tendon is usually a problem of overuse. Rest and cold the first day. Rest and heat over subsequent days.

Knee aches: usually torn supporting ligaments on the outside of the knee or structural ligaments inside the knee joint (the cruciate ligaments). Rest and cold on first day. Get professional help if not responding, especially if the knee gets puffy. It is a very vulnerable joint, especially if you are bringing an old injury to a new fitness program. Toning up the leg muscles may reduce joint 'wobble' and subsequent aching pain.

Hip injury: considerations here are similar to those for the knee. Early on, rest and hot bats. Get professional help regarding hip problems early rather than late.

Lower backache: usually complicating a racket sport or activation of an old contact injury. Rest and cold first day. Rest and heat thereafter. Professional help is a very reasonable move if walking brings on lower back pain. Consider a program of back strengthening exercises. The average American back is very vulnerable from a lifetime of physical inactivity and sitting at desks. Our back muscles are wasted. The two muscles that run down your back on either side of your spine should be as well developed as your forearm. Have a look in the bathroom mirror.

CHAPTER 4

YOUR OWN HELPING HANDS: DOWN OVER THE MONTHS

STEP 1

STEP 2

STEP 3

STEP 4

Most people who lose weight, studies show, gain it back within a year. Your body has begun to work against your best intentions. It is a creature of hard times and has gone into survival mode, slowing your metabolism and sending out hunger hormones.

"You mean a whole watermelon?" the husband had asked in disbelief, "a 20-pound watermelon?" The doctor nodded. He had come back to be sure, after hearing from his wife in the waiting room, that she was to fetch and eat a watermelon. During her office visit the doctor had pointed out how weight-controlling whole food could be, rather than doing her usual calorie counting. She questioned him about melons, having heard they were nothing but sugar and water. The doctor was re-assuring. They bought a watermelon on the way home, a 23-pound monster, the biggest on display, and she ate it all – 5 pounds a day on 4 different days– for a filling, appetite-satisfying, weight-controlling experience. Both were pleased. Thirty pounds of appetite satisfaction had produced no weight gain. That's one secret of weight control. Whole food. Unprocessed. Simple. Fresh or Microwaved from frozen.

Televised foods taste better than any food in history, thanks to the diligence of processing chemists and teams of flavor experts. But they do not satisfy the appetite. Feeding studies have shown that today's food items, with their emphasis on fats and oils, salt, sugar and refinement, must be eaten at levels of 3000 calories a day for full appetite satisfaction. The same experiments showed that traditional whole foods provide appetite satisfaction on an intake of only 1500 calories a day.

It is partly an effect of the fiber in whole food. Fiber is food residue. It provides no calories and consists of anything left over after normal digestion is complete. One way that it functions in appetite satisfaction is by holding water and bulking up food in the stomach. A pound of food fills most of us to satisfaction and signals the brain that enough is on board. A pound of oranges for example, will stretch the stomach at a cost of about 200 calories. A pound of chocolate does the same at 10 times the calories. The difference between oranges and orange juice is real. A couple of oranges satisfy the appetite for several hours, but de-fibering them (squeezing their juice into a glass) satisfies the appetite for barely and hour. See for yourself by trying it.

Do not be impatient with your body. It has thousands of years of history within its tissues. Slow and steady makes for habits that maintain your weight loss. A pound a week is a real progress, and regular exercise helps keep it off. People who maintain lost weight have been found to exercise for at least an hour most days. Cutting calories gets the weight down, but the portion control and fitness keep it there.

Let's say you've lost 25 pounds, and like the way you look and feel. Perhaps you're pleased you've lost the high blood pressure or blood sugar. Now, however, you've got 25 pounds of empty storage space (millions and millions of fat cells) open for business and waiting to be refilled. They are another reason why it is so easy to regain lost weight. It takes about five years for the empty storage space to totally close down. Early years of weight maintenance depend upon keeping those empty cells, empty. That is the reason for the Fist-of-Food approach.

Simply Tasty Fists Of Food

MICROWAVED POTATO & ONION, CHUNKED WITH
NON-FAT MAYO, SLICED GREEN BEANS WITH SLIVERS
OF TOASTED ALMONDS, EGG-WHITE OMLET WITH
MUSHROOMS & SPRINKLED PARMESAN, A MICROWAVED
YAM SPOONED OUT WITH TIPS OF NON-FAT MAYO,
MICROWAVED BRUSSELS SPROUTS KISSED BY DIJON
MUSTARD, NAVEL ORANGE SEGMENTS WITH AN OAT
& HONEY GRANOLA BAR, FRESH APPLE SECTIONS
DOLLOPED WITH PEANUT BUTTER, FRESH BERRIES
'CREAMED' IN A THICK VANILLA PROTEIN SHAKE, ANY
ASIAN DISH OF SEASONED RICE AND VEGETABLES

**AVOID BREADS AND WHEAT PRODUCTS.
THEY OFTEN ROIL THE APPETITE.
USE RICE, BEAN AND OAT PRODUCTS.**

The fitness minute involves calories expended in one minute of action, and used to balance calories taken on as special treats. A fitness minute takes your warmed up heart rate to 100-120 beats per minute, without discomfort, and holds it there for one minute. It could be scrubbing floors or garden chores; running, jumping, bicycle pumping; being in the swim, at the gym; dancing, prancing even heavy romancing. It burns 10 calories in a minute. By dividing the calories of any food item such as a double dip ice cream cone, by 10, you can translate the calories into necessary effort. An ice cream cone at 300 calories costs 30 minutes. A large apple at 80 calories costs 8 minutes. There are two budgets to weight control, and both must be balanced.

Tasty Stir-Fries For Two

At cooking time, heat splashes of oil, stock and sherry in a skillet at the highest setting. Add vegetables . . . two cups cleaned, trimmed and thinly sliced. (Cheat with frozen.) Toss and stir until tender/crisp: not over-cooked. Remove with a slotted spoon. To the liquid in the skillet, add 1/3 cup chicken stock. Simmer over low heat, until slightly thickened. Return vegetables to skillet and heat through. Serve over rice. Soy sauce it.

Suggested Vegetables – Fresh Or Frozen –

Carrots, celery, green peppers, scallions, cauliflower, cabbage, snow pea pods broccoli, mushrooms, bokchoy, zucchini, brussels sprouts, bean sprouts, bamboo shoots.

It is almost impossible to gain or lose a pound of fat in a single day. The bathroom scales measure body juices too, which can go up and down by 5 to 10 pounds in a day. Weigh yourself weekly and rely on clothing fit to keep you informed, fat-wise, or how about a fine gold chain snug against the skin around your waist? Diuretics (chemicals that prevent the kidneys from retaining water, the normal job of kidneys) interfere with this function and cause water loss and weight loss. Other fluid accumulations and weight swings can result from: allergies, the menstrual cycle, and food sensitivities. They bloat the face in the morning, make finger rings snug, and cause feet and ankles to be puffy through the day.

BE SURE TO READ CHAPTER FOURTEEN

CHAPTER 5

YOUR OWN HELPING HANDS: INDEPENDENT AT A HUNDRED

STEP 1

STEP 2

STEP 3

STEP 4

STEP 5

A Lifestyle: New Ways For New Weighs

To celebrate its own hundred years of existence, the National Institutes of Health did a survey some time ago, of hundred-year-old citizens, asking them to account for their longevity. To what habits or practices did they ascribe their long lives? It was a waste of public money, but among the more entertaining explanations recorded: a daily pinch of snuff, a daily verse of Scripture, regular shots of whiskey, a daily bowel movement, a cup each day of camomile tea, a glass of dandelion wine, and on it went. Most of those interviewed were stick-thin and had lived hardscrabble lives. They had known a time before automobiles or airplanes, television and electronics. They had also lived through two World Wars, and a Great Depression. Most confided that they would rather not have to go through it all again, thank you.

Sugar Into U.S. Food Supply per Person Per Day

1970 350 calories 1980 400 calories

1990 450 calories 2000 475 calories

2010 475 calories

If you want to stay lean and live an independent, pleasant life to 100 years, you will have to change your habits, not just for an ideal weight, but for a vigorous and independent hundred years. It's your choice, because as soon as you stop 'dieting', old habits will return you to where you were when you started this trip. Staying at an ideal weight is not a diet but a way of living, a lifestyle. Daily walks cut the risk of heart attacks in half, lift the mood, promote a sense of well-being, tone up muscles, reduce irritability and sleeplessness. In brief, they improve every aspect of your mental and physical condition.

Let your fist be an ever-handy guide to portion control. Fill an imaginary rice bowl with vegetables made delicious by stir frying or with seasoning. Use meat or fish in chunks no longer, but slivers for flavor and textural interest. Indulge yourself in foods you enjoy, or you will feel deprived and less inclined to a healthful foodstyle. Half of each meal should be vegetables. An easy mantra you should commit to repetition: *Daily: five fruits, five vegetables, five miles.* There is no room in such a lifestyle for fast foods, sandwiches, deep-fried items of any kind or meals in a box handed to you through a drive-by window. In restaurants, share those oversized portions, so routine on every plate, with a dining friend.

CRAVINGS CROPPERS

as appropriate, to stop a craving try:
ONE SERVING OF A 'LIQUID PROTEIN' MILK SHAKE
LARGE CRISP DILL PICKLE
FORKFUL OF PEANUT BUTTER
TEASPOON OF DRY COCOA POWDER
TABLESPOON OF CLOVER HONEY
SECTIONS OF NAVEL ORANGE WITH OAT & HONEY
GRANOLA BAR
A SALTED CELERY STALK / CARROT STICK
HOT BOWL OF BROWN RICE, SOY-SAUCED
DEVELOP ONE OF YOUR OWN

SOME GOLDEN HABITS FROM MY BEST GOOD LOSERS

Clear out of your presence *EVERYWHERE* all packaged snacks and sweets.

Tell any friends you are on a program, *NEVER* a diet.

Dress for success with fetching workout shoes and sportswear.

Work out with a friend at least once a week. It will keep you both obligated.

Keep tasty vegetables cut, clean and ever-ready in any fridge you may get near.

At restaurants: split food items

Stay away from buffets. You'll be too tempted to get your money's worth.

For neighborhood potlucks, take a shrimp platter and eat from it.

Good restaurants post menus online. Check ahead to order sensibly.

Wear a fine gold chain monitor, snugly around your newly-narrowed waist.

A SUCCESSFUL RETIREMENT BEGINS EARLIER THAN MOST PEOPLE REALIZE.

Connecting The Dots . . . To A High Blood Cholesterol

EVEN THE SMALLEST BUBBLE BELLY . . .

. . . floods the liver with fatty acids,

. . . that slowly choke important machinery in liver cells,

. . . and allow excessive bad cholesterol into the circulation,

. . . which gets under the linings of the body's arteries,

. . . and collects in lumps like limestone in a water pipe,

. . . to reduce blood flow to the legs and heart and brain.

CHAPTER 6

FRESH INSIGHTS. . . INTO METABOLISM

Summary

Metabolism is the process that maintains conditions in the body essential to life. It includes all life's chemistries, the sum of interactions that balance the energy and nutrient needs of each living creature, plant or animal, so it can live and thrive.

Metabolism preserves during life the delicate balance between too little and too much from moment to moment: keeping each organ system on track, while contributing to the needs of all other body parts.

One piece of folklore a doctor acquires with any European patient contact, is the national organ focus: Germans, for example, feeling out of sorts are inclined to blame their stomachs, the British their bowels, and the French, their livers. New findings from research into metabolism over the past decade should incline Americans, like the French, to blame much ill-health on their livers, It is Supreme Headquarters for the mischief created by our bubble bellies, our toxic waists.

Metabolism involves the chemistry of life. It includes the conversion of food and nutrients into products called metabolites for incorporation into tissue building blocks, converted to other products, or reduced to energy, carbon dioxide and water. Metabolism is mostly concerned with the needs of life so that living creatures have the energy and inner health to thrive in their environments.

In normal cells, such as those of liver or muscle, metabolism is highly organized and dynamic. Moment to moment, cells regulate and distribute needed nutrients and energy. They 'twitter' each other constantly, electrically or chemically, sending out steady streams of signals that keep everything synchronized and working to the body's overall benefit. Metabolism is the process by which we find and use energy, find and use tissue building blocks, locate damage and begin repairs. All this activity depends on oxygen, whose consumption is called The Metabolic Rate. Exercise experts use it to improve the performance of athletes.

The Portal Vein carries products of what we eat and digest to the liver to be sorted, and sent on their way in the circulation as metabolites to all parts of the body.

Proteins are construction blocks for body cells and for items like genes and enzymes. Proteins take longer to digest and some of their constituent amino acids have a suppressing effect on appetite. The popular protein milkshake is effective in this regard but no more than 3 should be taken in any 24-hour period. Too much protein, to the exclusion of carbohydrate and fat, risks other health problems.

Carbohydrates are spooled sugars, hence the name: complex carbohydrates. They are the prime components of foods like potatoes, rice, breads and pasta.

Fats and oils give food a rich and creamy mouthfeel. They help achieve a sense of fullness, but are calorie bombs and loaded with energy. Fats and oils require no biochemical conversions in the body. They are burned as fuel or stored as future fuel or incorporated directly into the walls of tissue cells, so eventually you become what you eat . .

. trans fats, saturated fats and all. The American diet is over-rich in fats and oils.

U.S. FAT&OIL CONSUMPTION

1950   300 calories per day

1960   350 calories per day

1970   400 calories per day

1980   425 calories per day

1990   450 calories per day

2000   600 calories per day

2010   650 calories per day

Trace nutrients once meant vitamins and minerals, but new research provides insights into other functions. Trace nutrients help prevent cancer (as antioxidants) and some have other therapeutic benefits. Isolated into capsules and bottled, they are being called nutraceuticals, but all their benefits are available in whole foods, which is a good reason for shifting to that dietary preference.

Food fiber is indigestible food residue. It does not get into the Portal Vein but remains behind in the intestines. It holds water, captures and carries away natural food toxins and contributes to the ease with which you move your bowels.

The Pancreas is an abdominal organ that plays an important role in digestion, producing and delivering powerful enzymes into the digestive tract. The pancreas also makes insulin, a hormone released into the Portal Vein that flows to the liver. One of insulin's roles, once through the liver and out into the general circulation, is to stimulate the distribution of selected nutrients into tissues of the body.

Insulin sends amino acids into cells. It sends a rising blood sugar into muscles and fat stores. High insulin levels, however, when sustained over time, are not good for us. They alter several metabolic balances in the body. *Because insulin retains salt,* high levels lead to an elevated blood pressure. *High levels also promote cancer.* Insulin does not cause cancer but present in high levels, helps promote its growth. Cancer researchers demonstrated decades ago, that animals inoculated with cancer cells survived longer if placed on semi-starvation diets after inoculation. Such diets kept the cancer animal's blood insulin levels low.

Other cancer researchers confirmed that for cancer cells to grow in culture, insulin and sugar must both be in the nutrient broth. Normal cells grow without insulin in the broth. Over the next few pages you will find illustrated some explanations of how current scientific understanding of the bubble belly acting upon the liver becomes a toxic waist, to produce most of today's lethal diseases. Study them carefully and realize the extent to which heart attacks, strokes and cancer are now understood to be self-inflicted wounds.

The Major Players In Today's Killer Diseases

CHOLESTEROL MOLECULES
Made in liver / present in diet / delivered into blood

BLOOD SUGAR MOLECULES
Made in liver / present in diet / delivered into blood

INSULIN MOLECULES
Made in pancreas / delivered into liver and
small amounts released into blood

FATTY ACID MOLECULES
Delivered to liver in diet
Delivered to liver by visceral fat (Bubble Belly fat)

Fat's most conspicuous collections in normal adult bodies are around the hips and belly. Young women normally lay down fat in the breasts and hips at puberty. Belly fat is the typical male distribution laid down later, and the two collections behave differently: abdominal fat is more active, meaning it has a rapid turnover of its constituent fatty acids compared to the more sluggish turnover in pelvic (hip) fat.

Fat around the abdomen (See diagram) drains directly into the liver through the same vein that drains the pancreas, the abdominal organ that produces insulin. The steady flood of fatty acids from a big belly into the same vein transporting insulin interferes with the liver's normal uptake of the insulin. More escapes into the blood where it raises the blood pressure, later the blood sugar and then the susceptibility to cancer, all cancers.

A recent British report emphasized how the *abdominal fat* of the bubble belly is associated with more cancer in women than is fat around their hips. From 2000 to 2010, they followed death rates in the U.K. from cancer of the uterus. Death rates doubled over the decade, closely associated with bubble bellies rather than broad hips. Belly fat is the new focus of clinical attention, with its insulin connection.

Overwhelming The Liver's Metabolism:

The diagram above illustrates how large collections of abdominal fat load the liver with fatty acids and overwhelm its capacity to keep the body's metabolism normal. Cholesterol escapes to clog the arteries. Insulin escapes to raise the blood pressure. High levels of insulin eventually induce tissue resistance to its action, produce 'insulin resistance' and the elevated blood sugar of diabetes. High and sustained circulating insulin levels heighten susceptibility to cancer. Finally, the latest piece of bad news: fatty acids eventually choke the liver into the inflammation and scarring of cirrhosis. Specialists in Digestive Diseases predict that the most common cause of cirrhosis will soon be the bubble belly. It is truly a *toxic waist*.

Cancer susceptibility has now been studied in patients with diabetes, the common overweight type that responds to oral agents. One drug used to treat them raises insulin levels. In long term studies it has been found to be associated with more cancers than another diabetes drug that lowers sugar by a different mechanism. Large and controlled trials are now underway to confirm or refute these early observations. As presently understood, elevated insulin levels set the stage for whatever type of cancer might otherwise reflect one's gender (breast, prostate) or lifestyle (alcohol, smoking). Insulin does not cause cancer but facilitates its growth.

LIFE IS NOT SIMPLY ABOUT ENJOYING ONESELF
AND HAVING FUN. IT CARRIES PURPOSES
OF SURVIVAL AND REPRODUCTION,
PLUS THE SOCIAL & MORAL
RESPONSIBILITY
TO CONTROL ONE'S APPETITES.

CONNECTING THE DOTS . . .
TO A HEART ATTACK

EVEN THE SMALLEST BUBBLE BELLY . . .

. . . floods the liver with fatty acids,

. . . that slowly choke important machinery in liver cells,

. . . and allow excessive bad cholesterol levels into the circulation,

. . . which get under the lining of heart and brain arteries,

. . . and narrow irregularly heart artery tunnels,

. . . to reduce blood flow then plug up into a HEART ATTACK.

MEDICAL EMERGENCIES TAKE YEARS TO HAPPEN.

CONNECTING THE DOTS . . .
FROM BUBBLE BELLIES TO LETHAL DISEASE
OVERLOADED FAT CELLS CHOKE AND DIE

. . . to flood the liver with inflammatory products,

. . . that react with liver cells,

. . . creating a fatty, inflamed state,

. . . spilling products into the blood causing aches and pains,

. . . and leave a scarred, shrunken liver of HEPATIC CIRRHOSIS.

THE BUBBLE BELLY, *AT THE BASIC SCIENCE LEVEL,*
IS TIED TO . . .

HIGH BLOOD PRESSURE FOR **STROKES**

HIGH BLOOD CHOLESTEROL FOR **HEART ATTACKS &
   STROKES**

HIGH BLOOD SUGARS FOR **DIABETES**

HIGH BLOOD INSULIN LEVELS FOR **CANCER**

AND THE SCARRED, FATTY LIVER OF **CIRRHOSIS**

CHAPTER 7

FRESH INSIGHTS . . .
INTO TISSUE HOUSEKEEPING

Summary:

It is not dangerous to feel hungry, but essential to full health. Hunger is a sign that the cells of your body are performing their routine tasks of housecleaning: Called **autophagy**. *It is a fascinating process – only of late, well understood – whose failures are lethal and whose functions you can enlist to your benefit.*

Pronounced: 'otto - fa - jee', the word translates as self-digestion but we have learned that this one particular function is only part of its action. Autophagy does involve self-digestion, of damaged cell parts being repaired or replaced. Every one of the billions of cells in your body during times of hunger, when internal energy levels fall, first looks to energy resources within itself, energy it needs to maintain metabolism.

A cell consists of a nucleus (home of its genetic control system) suspended in a bath of thick surrounding juice called cytoplasm or cytosol. Out in the cytosol and waiting in suspended animation during the day (during times of nutrient abundance), waits the orchestra conductor of autophagy. The normal human cell works mostly during daylight hours, whatever its tasks in the body. Whether liver, kidney, brain or muscle, it works best during light time and rests for repairs during night time. We are not creatures of the night but the day and the light. When autophagy begins naturally, during the night hours, an elegant and orchestrated ballet of stunning complexity takes place for a cell's housekeeping tasks, to gather up stray nutrients floating in the cytosol and burn them, along with cluttering trash.

When energy levels fall inside a cell – normally at night while resting – the autophagy orchestra conductor migrates from the cytosol into the nucleus and taps to attention at least 35 genes. The genes release messenger proteins that leave the nucleus and migrate into the cytosol on two complementary missions. One is to form *a collecting net*. The other is to create *a recycling center*.

The collecting net gathers up cytosol particles of potential energy . . . sugars, fats, amino acids. It sweeps up useless debris from the cell's workday world of litter (bent and broken bits of cell machinery).

The collecting net's molecules, having migrated out from the nucleus into the cytosol, position themselves to form a net and get to work. Because they distribute themselves throughout the cytosol, they are called ubiquitins. (Who said scientists have no way with words?) On signal, the ubiquitin molecules link up with each other, form the net that sweeps up cell bits (called cargo) then head for the recycling center. The fused net and recycling center convert cargo into: energy, new building blocks and waste products like carbon dioxide and water.

The recycling center, the second messenger mission, becomes a powerful little digestion site, packed with strong oxidizing enzymes, and the actual place of autophagy. It will receive material collected by the net and once that job is done, will self-dismantle. The name of the center is the *lysosome.* Its working destiny is to fuse with the net, accept its cargo, then create energy and recycle usable parts. This is autophagy as currently understood. It takes place when you feel hungry, a signal that the cells of your liver and brain are doing some housecleaning, tidying up clutter that gums up cell machinery and interferes with full performance.

Changing weighs begins with an understanding of how the body works – like autophagy – then re-ordering one's habits in ways that go with the grain of your biology rather than disrupting and cutting across it. Analyze your food habits and lifestyle with an eye to identifying disruptors . . . your associates, your situations, your days. Once recognized, figure out new and better habits. You'll not change the world, only your way of living in it.

If work and obligations are not balanced by compensating breaks and rests, you will turn to the comfort of food and drink. The habit will eventually impact on your weight and will cost you your health. Today's favorite escapes are watching while eating over-salted, over-sugared, over-fatted and over-refined foods. They are flavorful but lack satisfaction as studies with oranges and apples have shown. Juice from the fruit (containing all the calories) satisfies for half as long as the fruit does. Real food, whole food, requires chewing, prepares the stomach, and delivers a stomach-distending package of nutrition in a slow and natural way over the hours.

Enjoy the company of friends over coffee, tea or ice water. Become aware of the social influences on your eating. Atlanta researchers persuaded 68 adults to maintain diaries of everything they ate or drank and the circumstances. The number of people with whom each ate was positively correlated with the amount of food each consumed. In the presence of others, even when not hungry, test subjects ate more food. Social factors increase food eating.

For many individuals food cravings begin late in the day when body tissues naturally want to tidy up. Most of the day's chores are done, you're tired and your guard drifts down. the market economy sees an opening. Food is a comforting approach but there are better alternatives: Take a powder . . . get on the treadmill, go for a hike, find a quiet place, meditate, nap, offload. Take a fancied powder . . . a scoop of protein powder in a bowl of skim milk with berries or chunked fresh fruit, the high-tech alternative.

In a world of abundance, such as ours, critical cellular housecleaning functions fail. Cells become cluttered and dysfunctional with junk. Over the decades we sicken and age prematurely. Pharmaceutical researchers are working diligently for agents that will activate the orchestra conductor of autophagy but why wait? Take a walk when hungry to get the process going. Even a small bubble belly leads to early declines in physical and mental ability.

People in retirement communities have repeatedly discovered how daily exercise improves their memory, their mood and sense of self-esteem. You might call it an anti-aging habit – a rejuvenator activated by the simple strategy of stepping out each day, perhaps to music.

Laboratory mice help explain some brain benefits beyond autophagy. The hormone of exercise is adrenaline, and when brain slices are incubated in it, their brain cells are stimulated into greater activity and growth. Exercise activates them. Patients with Alzheimer's or Parkinson's disease can slow the decline and improve their stability and balance. A mouse model has been genetically engineered to mimic features of Alzheimer's disease. When exercised, its muscles release another newly-discovered metabolite that clears vulnerable nerve cells of several Alzheimer's fingerprints.

ONE NEUROLOGICAL SIGN OF AGING IS THE SPEED AT WHICH NERVE PULSES ARE TRANSMITTED.

MEN IN THEIR 70S AND FIT FOR A DECADE, HAVE REACTION TIMES THAT ARE FASTER THAN MEN IN THEIR 40S WHO ARE SEDENTARY.

CONNECTING THE DOTS . . . TO A HIGH BLOOD SUGAR

EVEN THE SMALLEST BUBBLE BELLY

. . . floods the liver with fatty acids,

. . . that slowly choke important machinery in liver cells,

. . . and allow excessive insulin into the circulation,

. . . which provokes sugar-loaded tissues to block its effects,

. . . eventually leading to a state of insulin resistance,

. . . and raising the blood sugars to DIABETES MELLITUS

CHAPTER 8

FRESH INSIGHTS . . . INTO ENERGETICS

Summary:

The basic unit of human mobility is walking. Herein a review of the cellular and tissue basis of fitness and many of its documented benefits.

Few of us realize how costly it is to be a warm-blooded creature, how much food we need, say in excess of cold-blooded creatures, to survive and thrive. Being warm-blooded requires about 1,000 calories a day. The furnace that keeps us warm (our metabolism) needs a steady fuel supply to hold temperatures around 98 degrees Fahrenheit for every minute of our programmed 100-hundred years of life. Several degrees above or below is lethal. Keeping us warm is a major responsibility of what we eat, because in our dim and distant past it had survival advantages.

Being warm-blooded made us quick, compared to reptiles who function between wide ranges of body temperature, and the price they pay is low gear mobility. Their temperatures correspond roughly to their environment with a performance that varies accordingly. Warm-blooded critters such as we, live independently of such constraints. It had a major survival advantage, and its body-brain connection has placed us in charge of the planet.

For most of human existence, the daily muscular demands of several thousand calories accounted for the other calories we consumed: going about the daily business of finding our dinner without becoming someone else's. The physical exertion required for food and shelter these days ranges from 10 to 500 calories. *It is the reason why neither at home nor at work can we expect to use enough muscle power to keep us fit and well.* It must be at play. In an age of quick convenience our stone age bodies must have recreational effort that makes us put out at least 500 calories of effort a day.

Even a few minutes of daily walking strengthen our muscles and bones, promote self-confidence, relieve stress and help control weight. We have been walkers for a million years. Having mastered its basics in the first two years of life, it requires no special equipment or training. It is safe and available year-round, and out of the weather where shopping malls open early just for walkers. It is a natural tranquilizer, quite sociable, and effective for anyone wanting to be fit. Walking is the basic unit of human effort.

Six hundred California men and women who had successfully lost weight were evaluated 3 years later, to discover what habit change had lead to long-term success. All 600 initially lost to within 10 pounds of ideal. All were short-term successes. The difference between long-term success and failure, the researchers discovered, was a continuing fitness program. How they lost weight did not make a difference . . . whether doctor supervised, in a group, or done for medical or cosmetic reasons. The only assurance of long-term weight loss was fitness, and the minimum effective amount they found was half an hour 3 times a week. Any physical effort taking your heart rate above 100 beats a minute and holding it there, is a fitness activity. How times have changed.

If we share any regular physical activity today with our friends or work associates, it is watching superb athletes compete from our seats in the stands or from home on television. We are quite comfortable watching and munching, thank you, while heartily endorsing their athletic feats as a skill we much admire.

Although rarely regarded as a workout (because it seems so casual) walking can be aerobic. At a pace of one mile in 15 minutes, benefits begin although with little weight loss. At 5 miles an hour, walking burns calories in a weight-losing manner. It means a brisk and purposeful pace some call Power Walking. It changes the tempo and involves posture, arms and legs. Stretch and bend the joints in your hips and legs and shoulders for a minute or so before heading out.

Keep an upright posture for aerobic walking, eyes on the far horizon to bring your chin up and draw your shoulders back. Swing the arms forward from your sides so they help pull the legs along. Make your legs take faster, not longer strides. Imagine you are showing the sole of your push-off shoe to someone following. That mental picture will keep your trailing foot on the ground a millisecond longer for shorter, stronger, faster steps. Take your time getting down to 12 minute miles . . . at least a month.

Exercise produces brain and body benefits through the cellular housekeeping process called autophagy, described earlier. When available fuel falls within a cell, as during fasting or exercise, it begins to gather up loose bits of sugar and fat to burn, as well as any cluttering pieces of worn-out machinery. Such 'housecleaned' cells work better, and collectively, they function better. Their owner feels invigorated. It is a natural process that can be initiated anytime with a brisk walk, especially when hungry.

Both Fred Rollingstone's sons went to medical school. (You will meet the Rollingstone family in Chapter 12). The older one, more outgoing and decisive, pursued an interest in surgery – cardiac surgery – which became his specialty during Residency Training. He made a fine living performing coronary artery bypass grafts over the early decades of his career, while his younger brother regarded the procedure skeptically. The arteries being operated upon were diseased along their entire lengths, not just at the site being bypassed. He was the scholarly one, and enjoyed the challenge of basic medical science. He became a cell biologist after medical school, getting prestigious training out-of-state, and returned to his alma mater to teach physiology.

Over the years, both brothers gained weight. At family gatherings they would challenge each other over who had the smaller bubble under his belt, both admitting that it was an unwelcome trend. The younger one began to study exercise at the cellular level in his laboratory. He wanted to see if it had an effect on autophagy in the muscles of his mice.

The daily program of exercise he crafted for his mice involved placing each in in a beaker to tread water for increasing periods of time. Within days of the conditioning program, their muscles had developed new engine parts in each cell. Previously tolerant of torn membranes and twisted organelles, the exercised cells removed and replaced damaged parts. Such rejuvenated muscle cells also proved to be more fuel-efficient at every point he measured.

Another mouse genetic strain, known to develop obesity and diabetes, became his second research interest when sister Pebbles showed an elevated blood sugar in her second pregnancy. After two months on his water bath program, all mice of the obese and diabetic strain lost their fat and their high blood sugars.

Muscles are hungry consumers of sugar, taking up more than 80% of any in a meal, and lowering the level of sugar in the blood to produce an insulin effect, without the use of insulin. Exercise conditioning in the diabetic mouse reversed its diabetes. He shared the information with Pebbles and she began the practice of daily walks with her toddlers.

Cell biologist friends showed in their own laboratories that exercised muscle releases a chemical signal to the body's fat stores, that muscles twitter fat stores about their energy needs. Naming the signal irisin, after the Greek messenger goddess Iris, they found it to be a protein molecule released by muscle that tells fat to start burning. They speculated that its original function (Chapter 12, our ancestral Flintstones) was a possible defense against the cold. Shivering is a muscular activity. By releasing irisin the shivering muscles helped early humans stay warm while they looked for a warmer temperature. The future of irisin as a treatment for obesity is being explored in research laboratories around the world. Meanwhile, a brisk walk gets the process going, sending your own irisin out to twitter your fat stores to get burning.

An Overview Of The Toxic Waist
The Bubble Belly As A Hockey Game:

First Period Of Play. . .

The flood of fatty acids from a bubble belly overwhelms the liver's ability to soak them up and they appear in the peripheral blood attached to cholesterol molecules. The compound is called Very Low Density Cholesterol, and popularly known as 'bad' cholesterol. It is the kind that collects in the walls of arteries and leads to heart attacks from a disease called atherosclerosis. Heart attacks are now everyday medical crises. They result from the threatened death of a segment of heart muscle due to sudden blockage of an artery. The underlying disease (atherosclerosis) was first described more than a hundred years ago by a German pathologist. He found small droplets, like wax from a candle, under the lining of the larger arteries of older individuals.

Cutting several open, he likened their color and consistency to the cooked oatmeal he ate that morning for breakfast. The Greek word for gruel is *atheros*, and because the deposits were projecting bumps into the artery tunnel, he added the suffix *oma*, as pathologists do when describing tumors. Thus did *atheroma* enter the medical vocabulary.

Older deposits of such material in large arteries attract hardened cradles of scar tissue containing flecks of calcium, hence: *arteriosclerosis*.

The higher the blood level of cholesterol the faster do atheroma form and grow. It now occurs in young people. Studies of American teenagers who sadly died in auto accidents, reveal early deposits of atheroma in their arteries. When combined with a high blood pressure, cholesterol deposition is speeded up by simple pressure dynamics. In this way, and over time, a high blood cholesterol and high blood pressure lead to blocked arteries in both heart and brain.

Second Period Of Play. . .

Insulin from the pancreas is normally kept at low levels in the general circulation by the liver. As the flow of fatty acids from a belly bubble increases, more insulin escapes into the general circulation and does two things: It sends sugar into the muscles, and it begins to raise the blood pressure (insulin is also a salt-retaining hormone). Elevated blood pressures respond nicely to a water pill or any one of a number of agents that relax the walls of smaller arteries. The latter work like nozzles in a garden hose, moderating blood pressures by moderating flow. Very high blood pressures can burst an artery in the brain and cause a stroke. It is called a hemorrhagic stroke because it bleeds into the brain, and is the most devastating type of stroke. There are two other kinds: thrombotic and embolic. Thrombotic strokes result, as in heart attacks, from a narrowing of the artery with cholesterol deposits to get plugged with a blood clot.

The third kind of stroke is a slap shot, occurring suddenly and unexpectedly, most often from a tiny clot forming in the heart. It gets loose in the circulation and lodges in an artery of the brain. This is the embolic stroke and often complicates an irregularly beating heart. Blood is delayed in the heart's upper chamber, 'puddles' during the delay and clots form. Blood not flowing briskly is liable to form clots.

During the Second Period, blood pressures are often high enough to excite clinical interest. It is a recognized health risk factor, and steps are taken to reduce it. Elevated pressures respond nicely to a water pill or any one of a number of agents that directly relax the walls of smaller arteries. An elevated cholesterol is often present, and sometimes in the company of another blood fat called triglyceride. The doctor may also prescribe a cholesterol-lowering agent.

Third Period Of Play. . .

Insulin resistance complicates the game in this period, as muscle cells resist the sugar-loading pressures of extra circulating insulin. Blood sugars drift up. Diabetes can be diagnosed with a sugar drink called the glucose tolerance test, and physicians often refer to a diagnosis at this stage as 'chemical diabetes'. Eventually the sugar goes high enough to spill into the urine. Patients are told to reduce their weight but the focus is more often on taking medications . . . for the sugar, the pressure and the cholesterol.

Later stages of diabetes have been recognized for centuries. Named diabetes mellitus by early physicians, they were describing what they found: They tasted the urine of patients complaining of thirst and urination, found it to be sweet, and called it the 'sweet pissing disease.' Hence *diabetes* (flow through) and *mellitus* (honey). It is never a sweet experience for the patient. High blood sugars glaze selected tissues in the body: the eyes (diabetic retinopathy), the kidneys (diabetic nephropathy) and the nerves (neuropathy).

Long-standing high blood sugars carry a delayed penalty. They lead to sugar-protein complexes that glaze the eyes, the kidneys and the nerves. Such glazing also accelerates the accumulations of atheroma in major arteries. Strokes and heart attacks commonly complicate the late diabetic life. Managing these problems calls for clinics and hospitals, for technical interventions and the skills of specialists.

CHAPTER 9

FRESH INSIGHTS . . . INTO HABITS

Summary:

We are all creatures of habit for good reason: They simplify daily decision-making. They are shortcuts to a purposeful activity that needs no thoughtful input. Thinking involves work, and habits provide the doing without the need for thinking. Habits are triggered by situations. By identifying the situation (1), then crafting another reward (2), you create the start of a new habit (3), to keep the lost weight off.

Habits are central to our market economy. Each television food commercial is intended to induce us to create a new habit, to eat a particular item and continue doing it: A skeptical celebrity (our stand-in) tries a new food and smiles re-assuringly. We are being taught a new food habit, assured by our celebrity stand-in, (a familiar cartoon character for kids). We associate the purchase with a reward. Like a laboratory mouse trained to press a lever for a food pellet we are conditioned by repeated viewings to begin pressing the lever. Millions of dollars are spent every day to shape our food habits. If each American were to eat just 500 fewer calories each day (the amount nutritionists calculate we eat in excess every day) it would cost the food industry billions of dollars a year. They will not take such a change in habit lying down.

Habits are housed in the most primitive part of the brain, a concentration of nerve centers that control other automatic functions of the body like breathing, digesting or the heart beat. Make a clenched fist. Your 'habits center' is about half that size but just as lumpy and located in the base of your brain. Think of it as Old Brain because we share it with creatures on the planet millions of years before we arrived. Old Brain is densely wired to New Brain, the cauliflower-like structure most of us visualize as The Brain.

New Brain grew up out of Old Brain, and is the home of our intelligence. It is where we figure things out, which is hard work. Old Brain works automatically. It works without thinking at effortless repetitive activities like breathing and heart beating, and on *habits,* as new research reveals. New Brain teaches Old Brain some new activity it has learned, then turns responsibility for performance over to Old Brain as a habit, for example: brushing our teeth or combing our hair. Such habits are useful and need no decision-making nor hard thinking. New Brain can then devote itself to what is happening around us. An estimated 40% of what we do each day is a collection of effortless habits.

New Brain explores the world around us, keeping us out of harm's way while daily routines become the job of Old Brain, the body's autopilot of easy habits. Think of them as apps of computer code, developed and inserted by New Brain to be activated by triggers for the reflex delivery of a rewarding action. You feel uncomfortable: angry, hungry or nervous. That is the trigger for a reward . . . a bite to eat. A cigarette. A beer.

The secret to permanent weight control is to analyze situations that trigger your feeding app, situations that prompt an urge to eat . . . Feeling lonely? Watching television? The office coffee break? Exhaustion from a tough day? An exasperating relationship? Once identified, you re-code your present eating response to trigger a new reward, a new habit that adds fewer or no calories without re-enforcing any other bad habit. Instead of the coffee with everything, coffee plain. Instead of the cruller with coffee you pull out a granola bar.

Alcoholics Anonymous is dedicated to changing alcoholic drinking habits. Millions of troubled individuals benefit every year from its famous Twelve Step Program. Most of the steps mention God or spirituality, and weekly support meetings encourage alcoholics to share their stories with other sober alcoholics, to stay away from situations that involve drink. When confronted by triggers with drink as the reward, participants develop escapes, other entertainments, some other release . . . new habits. They are provided a sympathetic ear in the sponsorship of a buddy. Alcoholics Anonymous provides an appropriate model for weight control, expecting all participants to substitute new and safer routines for old self-destructive ones. It succeeds best when participants "believe" in something: God for some; that things will get better, doing it for others, or simply . . . I am worth it!

Habits are not addictions but natural behavior shortcuts that evolved to save us from the hard work of thinking. They are useful. Craft new ones to your needs: a new routine in response to the familiar signal. Repetition will gradually groove it to a comfortable fit. Do not rely on willpower. You will be denying a behavior too hardwired from antiquity. Try not to eat while working, or sitting at your desk, or watching television or driving the car. Eating is a pleasurable experience to be enjoyed. Savor whatever food you do eat. Relax and focus on it. In the company of friends around food, have a cup of coffee or tea. Studies show that we eat twice as much in company we would if alone or at home. Begin to consume your calories on your own, while enjoying the company of others calorie-free.

Taking alcohol with food is a risk . It increases calorie consumption. Even when the beer is lo-cal, its alcohol tends to dissolve control. After indulging yourself in feast at a special event, get right back on track with a protein powder.

Some Simple New **Habits** To Consider

Take regular breaks, morning and afternoon. Pretend to be going to the bathroom if necessary, but start walking on breaks. Begin by using the stairs. You only need 15 minutes. Five miles a day are steps to a slimmer future.

Develop a support system of individuals who also want to get control of their weight. You'll discover neighbors, other workers or friends who will join for company.

Create a week-end fitness obligation with a friend . . . in the park or at the mall.

Turn off the screen for an hour every evening and pick up a book, listen to music, paint a picture, browse the neighborhood, get a dog to walk.

Learn to dance, to collect antiques, to be a good neighbor, a Good Samaritan.

Few things are more precious than our habits, embedded as deeply as they are in emotional Old Brain. They are comforting, powerfully anchored, viscerally defended and famously resistant to change. They have taken us time to develop, and a little daily dedication to keep polished. They make the tough patches in life easier and save us the hard work of decision making. They gratify cravings, get work done, relieve anxiety and make us feel loved. The easiest decision to make regarding a bubble belly is to look around and discover that everyone else has one, decide its normal, grab a slice of pizza, relax and enjoy the game. Habits define our lives and sadly our health.

Expect glitches and setbacks. Negotiate agreements with parties contributing to your predicament, but not in an angry mood. Develop some self-analysis: Tinker, modify, persist. You're looking for long term results. Today's health problems are habit problems, and programs rather than diets provide your way out. It takes time to change health-undermining habits but you will look better, feel better, function better and live better.

Market forces in a free society are powerful habit-formers. They condition us to sit, to eat and to drink. They push all our hot buttons (and in defiance of common sense) promise a carefree future where we zip around in a happy electric chair. At least once a week you'll be reminded that when a medical emergency strikes, you'll get the best of emergency attention from the caring health professionals at nearby *St. Swithin's General,* while the TV voice-over intones: *"Have You A Saint For A Doctor?"* In case you failed to notice, health care is a market force, too.

FIVE STEPS TO CHANGING HABITS

1. **TAKE INVENTORY OF YOUR ASSETS.
   DON'T OVERLOOK WHAT YOU ALREADY HAVE.
   SET REASONABLE GOALS AND WORK TOWARD THEM
   FROM WHERE YOU ARE.**

2. **START WITH WHATEVER IS EASIEST OR MOST
   AGREEABLE FOR THE QUICKEST RETURN ON YOUR
   EFFORT WHICH HELPS OVERCOME INERTIA.**

3. **DON'T RUSH TO GET IT ALL DONE BY TOMORROW.
   LIFE IS A PROCESS OF CHANGE AND BECOMING, AS IS
   HEALTH.**

4. **LEARN TO DO AS MUCH AS YOU CAN WITHOUT HELP.**

5. **LET FAMILY AND FRIENDS ENRICH YOUR LIFE. LET THEM IN ON YOUR PLANS AND PROJECTS. SHARE SOME SECRETS.**

CONNECTING THE DOTS . . .
TO CLASSIC SUGAR DIABETES
EVEN THE SMALLEST BUBBLE BELLY

. . . chokes the liver and allows excessive insulin to circulate,

. . . inducing insulin resistance, diabetes and high sugar levels,

. . . in a patient feeling tired until sugar levels spill in the urine,

. . . and provoke excessive urination, with thirst with weight loss,

. . . going on, if untreated, to drowsiness, coma and death;

. . . for the ancient 'Pissing Disease' of SUGAR DIABETES.

A decade of cellular research into inflammation and the bubble belly has been insightful. When overfilled fat cells choke to death and disintegrate, ancient defenses treat the disintegrating bits like invading bacteria. Inflammatory products circulate through the body, antibodies are created. The results are aches and pains and insulin resistance, expressed clinically as fatigue, ill health and diabetes.

CHAPTER 10

FRESH INSIGHTS . . . .
INTO THE 'SLOW METABOLISM'

Summary:

Metabolism begins a spontaneous and natural slowdown during the middle years, a time of life when most weight-prone individuals have lost weight several times. They starved themselves down, by simple calorie restriction and without significant exercise, losing **both fat and muscle**. *Loss of muscle further slows metabolism.*

Many patients do not lose weight on the traditional doctor/dietitian prescribed 1200 calories a day. They ascribe it to their 'slow metabolism,' and a few do have an underperforming thyroid gland. Most physicians check for this during their routine evaluation these days. Many such patients have been 'watching their weight' for years and most have lost a batch several times by limiting calories. It worked well initially: best the first time, but less and less effective thereafter.

Here is why: Inside each of our bodies (beneath the skin but outside the skeleton) lie two major organ systems. One generates energy and heat – the red muscle organ system. Even at rest, muscle fibers tighten and relax spontaneously during life, generating heat and burning calories. Exercise keeps them bulked up and turning over like the engines they are. The other organ system provides fuel but no heat – the yellow fat one. Under-water weighing reveals all as you will see, paragraphed below.

In a study of red and yellow organ systems, all participants were placed on a diet of 1000 calories a day. Half of them included a walking program that lasted 30 minutes each day. The other half did not but simply restricted their calories as a 'diet-only'. After two months, the 'diet-only' group averaged a weight loss of 20 pounds, whereas the 'diet-walking' group lost 23 pounds. On the face of it, not a very impressive benefit from the added walking: only 3 pounds! The walkers felt cheated. But all had been weighed under-water, which was most revealing.

Under-water weighing enables measurement of fat and muscle separately. The diet-walking group *gained* 2 pounds of muscle during the study, masking a total fat loss of 25 pounds. The diet-only group *lost* 8 pounds of muscle, and only 12 pounds of fat. On the surface both groups lost roughly the same, but had different outcomes under the skin. The diet-walkers *lost 25 pounds of fat, the diet-onlies 12 pounds of fat*. Their futures will be very different. The diet-only group will regain the lost fat easily, blame a 'slow metabolism' while failing to realize how their lost muscle mass contributed to the 'slow metabolism.' There is a slowdown of metabolism with age. Sometimes from a declining thyroid production, which may slide with age, but usually it's the natural decline in muscle mass, normally 1% per year after age 30. It can be slowed by exercise but not stopped.

It would be logical to use hormones such as adrenaline and thyroid for a 'slow metabolism', or drugs like ephedrine for their fat-burning benefits. Sadly, they overstimulate the heart and raise the blood pressure. They also lift the mood and patients risk becoming drug dependent, side effects that preclude any general application. Researchers are looking for drugs that will safely burn off fat and not cause other problems. Nearly 100 years ago, during the first World War, women began working in munitions factories. They began to inhale a chemical in the dust of explosives that they discovered kept them thin. Doctors started using it for weight control until all the patients developed cataracts. A safe and useful drug is needed because obesity has become a world-wide epidemic. Affluence and abundance are reaching millions of people in Asia and Africa. The lethal diseases of the toxic waist will overwhelm the finances of every healthcare system.

Finally, there is a bubble belly gender gap. Young women begin adding fat to their hips and thighs at puberty, not to their bellies, as a gift of Mother Nature. Women are different from men in their circulating hormones, in the number of calories they need to live, and in the way they use and store energy. Before puberty, girls and boys generally have little excess body fat, but after puberty girls carry 10-15% more, not of the dangerous kind. Mother Nature developed in them a safer defense against starvation in the interest of species survival. After the menopause, however, protection from the bubble belly disappears.

OUR BIOLOGY & INGENUITY ARE MISMATCHED.
WE HAVE ENGINEERED EXERTION OUT OF LIFE.

CHAPTER 11

WEIGHING IN . . .
HOW WE GOT HERE

Summary:

Hard as it is to accept, today's greatest threat to health is abundance: an abundance of food, and an abundance of ease.
We have been designed by Mother Nature for tougher times.

National statistics indicate that the average body weight of adult Americans has gone up by about 50 pounds in the past 50 years. The epidemic got firmly under way in 1980 and continues to this day to the point that more than 25% of young American recruits for military service are rejected for obesity.

AVERAGE U.S. BODY WEIGHTS

1950   140 POUNDS

1960   145 POUNDS

1970   150 POUNDS

1980   155 POUNDS

1990   160 POUNDS

2000   170 POUNDS

2010   180 POUNDS

Back in 1962, the US Coast Guard mandated that all ships ferrying passengers in American waters estimate the average passenger weight at 140 pounds. In 2012, they mandated a new estimated weights up to 180 pounds.

"Our ships' centers of gravity have gone up," explained the grinning Coast Guard officer while making his announcement. The rude truth is they were playing catch-up with the Federal Aviation Administration. A decade earlier the FAA increased passenger weight averages on winter flights to 195 pounds.

Food abundance began with the best of intentions in the 1930s, during the Great Depression when government policy encouraged corn production with financial subsidies. The depressed agricultural community was pleased. Corn offered many markets, both at home and abroad, but the subsidies continue to this day and have discouraged growth of other foods on millions of acres of land. The agribusiness came into existence with these inducements, specializing in the production of two or three products – called mono-crop cultivation – but especially corn. It was an immediate food with global appeal, and clever chemists would eventually convert corn into sugar, alcohol, fuel, paint, whatever . . . feeding any residue to cattle for what would become the nation's most popular meat dish, hamburgers.

US DRY CORN PRODUCTION
ANNUALLY IN TONS

1970 100 million

1980 125 million

1990 150 million

2000 200 million

2010 300 million

Food convenience began in California during the 1940s, when two New England brothers named McDonald developed a clean and speedy system for delivering hamburgers to people in their automobiles. They opened several places, and a milkshake-maker salesman from Illinois bought the business, took it national and then global. Similar ventures during the 1960s and 1970s proved successful for chicken and ethnic foods like pizza and tacos. We became a nation in love with the convenience of fast foods.

A hundred years ago, the Basic Four approach to a healthful diet was enshrined in nutrition teaching. It was a kind of instructional short-hand conveying the need for nutrient variety. The Four Food Groups consisted of 1) Dairies, 2) Meats, 3) Fruits & Vegetables and 4) Grains. Sadly it has become an approach that can make your very sick – aggravating hypertension (its salt) while sending blood grease levels up with cholesterol and saturated fat. Its creamy fat mouthfeel promotes cancer, while the loss of fiber leads to diverticulitis. New replacements for the Basic Four continue to be proposed by appropriate committees but so entrenched are market forces in our food supply that nutrition advisory panels proposing Pyramids and Dinner Plates are repeatedly frustrated in the interest of preserving the status quo.

Much of today's food has sacrificed the nutrition variety that once justified the Basic Four. An onion is nutritionally different from an apple, but the differences pale to insignificance when eaten as onion rings or apple fritters. They taste good, no one denies, but sick they are making us. No country in the world spends more on medical care (AKA Health Care) than we do, yet the citizens of other countries outlive us. They eat differently. They live differently.

Back when the Basic Four became our food guide, most people walked to work and labored there 10 hours a day, six days a week. Household chores also took 10 hours most days and involved much lugging. Glance at old photographs of holiday crowds or celebrating groups from those days and you can see the shocking extent of change in our corpulence. Labor-saving advances in the workplace and at home, and advances in the production and processing of food have eased the labor of our days. Who shovels coal, or lugs firewood, or hauls wet laundry out to a clothes line? Who cooks large meals like TV chefs? Food is marketed for microwaving. It has an agreeable taste, appearance, price and shelf life. It comes to us from around the world. Market forces are entwined with today's diet and today's diseases. We must begin to enjoy their welcome benefits without sacrificing our health.

US CHEESE CONSUMPTION
PER PERSON PER YEAR

1950 10 pounds

1960 12 pounds

1975 20 pounds

1990 25 pounds

2000 30 pounds

2000 600 CALORIES PER DAY

2010 650 CALORIES PER DAY

THE MARKET ECONOMY HAS A HUGE STAKE
IN KEEPING US JUST THE WAY WE ARE.

A trip down memory lane . . .

In the 1940s . . .

The Idaho potato displaced Maine as the pick of the crop.

In the 1950s . . .

A hamburger and fries became the trademark American meal.
New freezers and refrigerators at the grocer's and at home.

In the 1960s . . .

Coffee with cream and sugar 45 cals (**cappuccino now 140 cal's**).
Fast food items with bacon: 20%. (**now 70%**).

We like familiar brands, standard service, cleanliness and predictable items. We like the uniformity and absence of unpleasant surprises. Back when it began, there was a feeling of reassurance when traveling on summer excursions across the land over fast new Interstate Highways. Wherever we went on vacation the products ordered from familiar franchises were reassuringly the same.

Even when home, families began eating out more often, sometimes more often in a week than they ate food from their own kitchens. The youngest often selected where they would eat and usually it was for a toy premium. Beyond the political promise of a chicken in every pot, we also got a car in every garage which drew us to the suburbs. Well-maintained roads were lined by eating places that delivered quick and tasty food kept cheap by continuing farm subsidies for corn.

Those are the ingredients of today's obesity epidemic: an intersection of cultural, political, scientific and market trends. Each one an independent and laudable activity alone, they have acted in concert for the unintended consequence of today's ill-health, and threaten our prospects for tomorrow's potential as a vibrant nation.

Culturally we enjoy speed and convenience and meals that can be held in a hand. We accept food through a window and in a box. The foods we especially enjoy are ground meat, fried chicken and products made from corn. By subsidizing corn production we have produced cheap cattle feed, chicken feed and corn sweetener for soft drinks. This has kept food costs down to an astonishing extent. Scientifically, we have been able to produce hygienic, tasty and novel food products at only a slight cost in nutrient value.

Our lives have been enriched and eased by frozen fruit juice, TV dinners and modern supermarkets. No one is forcing us to sit and eat, yet that has happened increasingly over the past 30 years. There are no villains in the epidemic, just a combination of smart marketing to consumers who are innocent or indifferent.

Market forces have been effective in penetrating every organization and institution. Fast food folks target children especially with toys and games to establish long-term eating habits. The fast food kitchen behind the window or counter is not a kitchen, but the final distribution point of a very long and technically sophisticated food chain. The food that arrives at a franchise outlet is frozen, freeze-dried, canned or dehydrated from large production centers elsewhere in the country, or even across the globe. The obesity epidemic was not obvious for several decades, and it wasn't just the burgers and fries. It was serving sizes too.

Compare convenience foods then and now for portion size . . .

A three-inch bagel at 140 calories went to a six-inch bagel at 350 calories.

A 6 ounce soda at 85 calories went to a 20 ounce Big Gulp at 250 calories.

A 2.5 oz pkg of french fries (210 cals) to a 6.9 oz Big Bite at 610 calories.

A 1.5 ounce pizza slice (250 cals) to 'new-size toppings' at 425 calories.

US TV VIEWING
HOURS PER HOUSEHOLD PER DAY

1950 4.0 hours

1960 4.5 hours

1970 5 hours

1980 5.5 hours

1990 6.5 hours

2000 7.0 hours

2010 7.5 hours

FATS AND SUGAR ARE CHEAP AND FILLING.
THEY ARE THE NUTRIENTS OF POOR PEOPLE,
THE FATTEST AND SICKEST AMONG US.

We are creatures that emerged thousands of years ago into a world of scarcity. We survived by hard physical effort, taking huge risks and we prevailed. In our earliest emergence as recognizable human beings, we lived only long enough to raise the next generation. No female skeleton has been found from those ancient times, older than 30 years at time of death, and no male skeleton older than 40.

Life to our ancestors for hundreds of thousands of generations was nasty, brutish and short. The bodies they gave us handle abundance badly. They develop narrowed arteries, cancer and diabetes from which we die prematurely and expensively. Our health care costs are the highest in the world, approaching 20% of the national budget. We must get to know the animal within, its proper care and feeding. At any given food encounter we must begin to eat and drink no greater amount than the size of a clenched fist, and for the big 'grand' meal once each day, put both fists together and eat their combined volume. This practice will shrink your stomach down without surgery. It is never too late. Your ruins are still inhabited.

BEGIN TO REWARD YOURSELF WITH NON-FOODS. A BOOK.
NEW SHOES. A GADGET. SOME CLOTHES.
A DAY AT A SPA. HOW ABOUT A NEW CAR?

CONNECTING THE DOTS . . .
TO DIABETES AND ITS COMPLICATIONS

EVEN THE SMALLEST BUBBLE BELLY

. . . floods and chokes the liver with fatty acids,

. . . and allows excessive insulin to circulate

. . . inducing insulin resistance, diabetes and high blood sugar levels,

. . . which produce damaging sugar-protein complexes in small blood vessels,

. . . to effect the eyes, the kidneys, the nerves and larger arteries causing

. . . the blindness, uremia, and gangrene of DIAB. COMPLICATIONS.

CHAPTER 12

MEET THE STONES . . .
OUR TWO LEGACY FAMILIES

Summary:

Mother Nature's gift to women at puberty is fat around their hips and breasts. They are the more important gender for carrying our species into the next generation.

It is a legacy from times of scarcity and uncertainty. Stored fat is future energy.

It had and still has, survival value,

Meet The Stones

This is an account of two family legends: the Rollingstones who grew up in the suburbs of Mid-America in the 1950s and are all alive today; and the Flintstones who hunted and gathered for a living 25, 000 years ago. Their home was a cozy cave overlooking a fertile valley from halfway up the face of a protective cliff.

First, The Flintstones

Anthropologists tell us that the woman who modeled the 4-inch stone carving above, was one of our ancestral grandmothers. Hundreds of such figurines have been found across Europe from France and Spain to the Russian Steppes. They emerged at the end of the last Ice Age, and mark the beginning of our time. She was an important figure in her clan, a Headwoman who bore 5-10 children, only half of whom survived into adulthood.

She gave us our bodies and our brains. A recent analysis of 2000 skeletons from those times, reveal how we switched from hunting and gathering on the edges of receding glaciers to settled communities of farmers and herders; from life as nomads to life in and around urban centers. No adult from those most remote times lived beyond 40 years, so we are very much on our own after 40 when it comes to natural survival.

Now, The Rollingstones . . .

When Fred Rollingstone came home from the service, a job awaited him at the Ford dealership. He promptly married his childhood sweetheart, Wilma, who had captained the high school tennis team. She continued to work after the marriage, teaching elementary school, while they saved for a house in the suburbs. Times were good. America was in an optimistic mood. Friends were moving to California, but the Rollingstones were happy in the middle of the country where they raised a family of three children. Interstate highways and jet travel had come into their lives. They kept both friends and relatives within easy reach.

Fred was promoted to sales manager at the dealership, and Wilma stayed home to raise the children. They became a two-car family (the first on either side) and once their eldest reached 16, a three-car family. It made good sense. So many interests were scattered around town, and good roads lead everywhere. They also enjoyed the bounty of new labor-saving developments at home, work and play.

No longer were bread and milk delivered to the house. Tasty food was at hand 24-hours a day without even leaving the car, and they liked fast foods: the familiar brands, the clean, quick service and predictable flavors. They appreciated the lack of surprises wherever they traveled across the land. Reassurance awaited them at every franchised food stop.

As Headwoman of the Flintstone Clan she carried the tiny stone carving with her in a small leather pouch around her neck. It signified status. She was a celebrity. Her hair was thick and long, the yellow-tan color of ripened meadow grass, and she held it together behind her neck with a leather tie. Her facial features were small, sharply defined, and her eyes were blue. She had full breasts that remained uncovered indoors where she wore a leather skirt above her waist that she tied with a thong. Out in winter weather she wore a tunic, dressing for the cold with leggings that also tied around her waist. The winter tunic had a parka and no front opening. For special occasions she favored something longer, often elaborately decorated.

Food did not come easily to the Flintstones. Possessing only spears and clubs, they ambushed bison and mammoth for meat. The 'ready signal' would be waved to hidden chasers, who then leaped leap noisily into view of a grazing herd to stampede it toward the waiting ambushers – hidden around the mouth of a trap in a cliff opening, behind driftwood logs and heavy rocks. They could feel the drumming thunder coming. They could hear the bawling and grunting of panicked animals pierced by shouts and screams from Clan chasers, the lead bull galloping at full speed just ahead of a shaggy mass of huge horned animals into their trap.

Once inside and now aware of their plight, the bison milled about in noisy confusion. Ambush rocks and logs were heaved into place, and Clan members clambered in among the angry bellowing animals for the bloody job of hacking, thrusting and killing. They slit throats with sharp flint knives and drove hard-tipped spears deep into vital parts. It was extremely dangerous as the damaged creatures fought back, only to be struck or speared again and again, before staggering down to bleed to death. Paired teams of hunters rolled each one onto its back to expose the tender underbelly and slice it open. Intestines, stomachs and bladders were taken to a nearby stream for washing and rolling into compact balls, kept moist for days in the freshly stripped skins and later used. Some organ parts were for food, some became storage containers for water and oils, and some were dried to harden as net floats for the spring fish run. Little was wasted.

Each freshly killed carcass was cut into two hindquarters and two forequarters. The neck and midsection were cut in half. It all had to be carried home on Clan backs, usually two bundles to each carrier: one on a backboard and another atop the board, held in place by a tump line across the forehead. Properly packed, a strong adult Clan male could carry 200 pounds for 10 or 15 miles.

The knee joint of a bison or a mammoth was a favorite stew bone. Into the pot it went with vegetables, fresh in season or from storage baskets back in the cold cave. Their diet included groundnuts, wild carrots, a miscellany of roots and tubers or as well as the stems of swamp cattails and bullrushes. To thicken the stew, a mash of pounded grains was created from wild rye and barley. It needed salt which they added, and for a spicy flavor they crumbled in dried sage or mint or bitterroot onion. Kitchen work was hard and dangerous. It involved heavy lifting around open fires, and large hot stones dropped into woven pots of water. They pounded grains into cracked forms or into flour for baking tiny buns or thickening gruel. They mashed seeds into paste and collected cooking oil by pouring hot water over the mashed seeds. The oils floated up, were skimmed and saved.

As Headwoman our Venus was in charge of food and its preparation. She supervised the women who cooked and labored, and she benefitted from an excess food and ease in her position. She developed the bubble belly, immortalized in stone. Most of her children died young of infections – the diarrheas of infancy, and epidemics of diseases like measles, mumps or diphtheria. Most Clan members died in what we would now consider the prime of life: from childbirth, infections or injuries. We are their modern descendants but no smarter than they were. Our huge advantage is the long line of ancestors between us, ancestors who continued to accumulate knowledge and pass it on. They hunted and gathered to stay alive, developed and used stone tools. They left us graceful outlines of the animals they found around them, on the walls of their cave homes.

The day following any major Clan hunt a second group would go back for left over material cached under heavy rocks against the many watching and scavenging animals. Back in the lodge a grand feast and celebration would be enjoyed. Musicians would play, tapping notes out of animal ribs or skulls, drumming on skins stretched taut across deep pelvic bones and chanting traditional songs. There would be dancing around the hearth fire, and a lamp lit in thanksgiving before an ivory figurine of Earth Mother.

In the 1970s Fred sharpened his outdoor cooking skills, looking forward each season to their Saturday afternoon guests for grilled meat, bourbon and beer. They entertained neighbors and customers whom they carried with them in the move to a new neighborhood and upscale house in 1980.

By the time he was 31 years old, Fred Rollingstone had gained 15 pounds from his trim marriage weight. Wilma could not shed any of the weight she had gained around her hips and middle with the children. By the time she was 30, her slim figure had given way to an extra 30 pounds. Quitting smoking added more to both of them. Fred continued to develop his grilling skills, using the leanest of meat and a secret moistening ingredient, caramelized onions. The family ate out more often, sometimes several times a week, and Pebbles, their youngest, often determined where they went, usually for the toy premium.

All three Rollingstone children matured into fine young adults and attended college, the boys as medical students and Pebbles to graduate as an English Major. When Fred had his heart attack at 57 years of age, they blamed the stress of managing three dealerships. His surgeon son arranged for a coronary artery bypass at the Cleveland Clinic. Wilma's breast cancer was recognized early and removed, identified in one of her annual mammograms. Pebbles (now married and living across state) showed sugar in her urine during the second trimester of her second pregnancy. All family members, including both doctor sons had developed 'rounded figures'."It's in our genes," smirked the surgeon to his younger brother at one family Thanksgiving gathering, referring to their expanded waist lines."Tight jeans," agreed the younger brother, with a laugh.

WHEN TAKING CHARGE OF YOUR HEALTH,BEGIN BY LEARNING A FEWOF MOTHER NATURE'S RULES.

CONNECTING THE DOTS . . .
TO A (CLOTTING) STROKE . . .

EVEN THE SMALLEST BUBBLE BELLY:

. . . floods the liver with fatty acids,

. . . that slowly choke important machinery in liver cells,

. . . and allow excessive bad cholesterol levels into the circulation,

. . . which get under the lining of all arteries in the body,

. . . and form lumps that narrow irregularly the artery tunnel,

. . . to reduce blood flow before plugging up for a STROKE.

CHAPTER 13

WHAT'S EATING US . . .
PRESSING MEDICAL MATTERS

Summary:

The human body is tolerant of considerable neglect up to about age 40. Into the middle years and beyond, we are more or less on our own to develop heart attacks, cancer, strokes and diabetes. New science is showing us how to avoid them.

Heart attacks, strokes and cancer have been the leading causes of death in developed nations for more than 50 years. Slowly, piecing the data together like a great jigsaw puzzle, global research is providing ever more useful insights. For decades the heart attack emphasis has been cholesterol and diet. For the strokes or high blood pressure, doctors cautioned against salt and prescribed diuretics. For the blood sugar of diabetes – another epidemic of our time – there are oral medications, and for cancer: improved surgery, radiation and chemotherapy.

Recent fresh insights at the cellular level have disclosed how all these diseases relate to one another, and how the liver is at the center of this new understanding. It is being overwhelmed by a steady flood of fatty acids from the bubble belly, fatty acids that provoke high blood levels of cholesterol and insulin, and more mischief from there. With better understanding will come better management and superior outcomes, but today's prudent individual, who wants to live as long as possible while dying as young as possible, will begin new ways for better weighs.

Heart attacks continue to account for half of all adult American deaths, yet were rare in the early 1900s. Research first demonstrated how collections of cholesterol in artery walls underlay the clots that caused heart attacks. The collections came from cholesterol in the blood that came from food in the diet, and patients were advised to change what they ate to reduce blood levels: to eat less cholesterol and saturated fat. The Anti-coronary Club of New York, an association of patients was organized years ago to test the notion that lowering blood cholesterol levels by dietary means would be of benefit, and showed that it is. Other studies involving thousands of participants over several decades confirmed the findings: lowering blood cholesterol levels reduces the number of heart attacks.

Strokes are caused by an interruption of the flow of blood to part of the brain, not unlike a heart attack. The brain needs a blood supply – like the heart – but unlike the heart, the brain is not a tough muscle. It is made of soft, fatty material, and high blood pressures in such tissue can burst a blood vessel as another cause of stroke in addition to the blocking blood clot. Medical management of a high blood pressure targets salt in the diet and blood pressure drugs, and both strategies have reduced the incidence of strokes (and heart attacks).

Heart and brain arteries, by the time they plug with clot are stiff and inelastic. The normal problem arteries are soft, flexible and elastic, about as big around as a lead pencil. They are hollow tubes of muscle that work to deliver the heart's pumping outpourings, a recycled 3500 gallons of blood a day, along a delivery network that narrows down to the tiniest of blood vessels called capillaries. There are 400 miles of capillaries in each pound of flesh.

US MEAT CONSUMPTION
PER PERSON ANNUALLY

1950 450 pounds

1960 500 pounds

1970 550 pounds

1980 600 pounds

1990 625 pounds

2000 625 pounds

2010 650 pounds

A retired executive with summer and winter homes, was overweight in excess of 100 pounds, but proud of his clean coronary arteries. He kept angiograms at hand to prove it. Summer and winter he and his wife enjoyed ship cruises and the bounty of food they provided. Spring and fall the couple would enroll for a month at Duke University in the residential weight loss program. "Undoing cruise damage," they always grinned. Each of his surplus pounds added 400 miles of invisible piping that his heart had to serve until gradually it failed. He was on a heart transplant list and sleeping with oxygen at home, when it finally stopped, clean coronary arteries and all.

Traditional thinking on diabetes and obesity has been simplistic . . . that fat cells become overloaded and resist the insulin signal to take up sugar which then rises in the blood. It is the most common kind of diabetes, (Maturity-Onset, Type II) and for several decades doctors have advised weight loss while prescribing oral medications to lower the sugar. The name diabetes mellitus comes from medical antiquity. It translates as the 'sweet pissing' disease, because once the sugar rises high enough in the blood, some spills into the urine taking water with it to produce the classic symptoms of: thirst, urination and weight loss. Controlling those symptoms is easy. Preventing the later complications of diabetes is not easy. They result from sugar-protein complexes forming in vulnerable tissues and eventually damaging the eyes, nerves, kidneys and arteries. They form at blood sugar levels well below those spilling into the urine.

The association of cancer with excess weight has been recognized for decades, although the mechanism has been unclear until now. Obese patients have 34% more cancer than do non-obese controls. They also eat more fat. In Japan, one of the most notable food changes after 1950 has been an increased consumption of fats and oils. There are more meat and animal products in their diet, and a far greater use of vegetable oils for cooking. This change has been paralleled by a striking increase in deaths from cancer of the prostate among Japanese men, and cancer of the breast in Japanese women. High dietary fat intakes promote cancer.

Back in 1930, researchers using cancer-causing agents on the skin of test animals, found that the level of fat fed to the animal determined the ease with which cancer could be produced. The more fat fed, the more cancer. Similar studies on dietary fat have been made on mice and implanted breast tumors. When tumor tissue is transplanted into cancer-free mice, the implants grow best if the animal is on a high fat diet. Today's diet provides too much fat, in too many products. There's a teaspoon of oil in a cupcake, and 3 teaspoons of butterfat in a glass of whole milk. Few of us would add 12 teaspoons of butter to an 8-ounce baked potato, but that's what happens when potatoes become 8 ounces of potato chips. The fat is different, but the effect is not.

Cancer prevention begins by eating less fat, and continues by eating more fibered foods and more vegetables. Certain foods and nutrients have been found to have anti-cancer protective properties. High fiber foods are protective, as well as foods rich in vitamin A, or its precursor beta carotene, and vitamin C and vitamin E. Members of the cruciferous vegetable family (cabbage, cauliflower, broccoli and brussels sprouts) are especially cancer protective.

THE PROSPECTS OF CUTTING DOWN
ON MEATS AND FATS
PRODUCES A FLAVOR CRISIS IN MOST MOUTHS.

THE TOXIC WAIST OVER TIME . . .

Sketched above, are several decades in the life of a typical Toxic Waist. Its owner refers to it endearingly as his pot or paunch, while delivering an affectionate pat or caress. In its early years it's normal, they say. Perhaps the blood pressure is a doctor's first expression of concern. Alarm bells sound at 140/90: Essential Hypertension. Salt use is cautioned, medication prescribed and the bubble is ignored. Its normal, they say.

An aside, regarding clinical numbers. Mother Nature works on a gradient, but doctors prefer hard lines. Essential Hypertension exists at 140/90, and not 139/89. Average is what you find in any general population. Average goes up with age, and is *not* normal. *Normal* are the numbers carried by healthy young adults. Your normal weight is likely what you weighed at age 25. That's not normal, they say. Oh, but it is. With this in mind, here are some fasting and resting normal values . . . for blood pressure: 110/70, for a normal cholesterol: 150, blood sugar: 70, and resting pulse: 60 beats per minute.

GOOD HEALTH IS ABOUT NORMAL NUMBERS

GASTRIC BYPASS SURGERY IN AMERICA: PROCEDURES IN 2002: 50,000 IN 2010: 300,000. SURGEONS ARE NOW STOMACH STAPLING OBESE TEENAGERS.

CONNECTING THE DOTS . . .
TO A (BLEEDING) STROKE . . .

EVEN THE SMALLEST BUBBLE BELLY:

. . . floods the liver with fatty acids,

. . . that slowly choke important machinery in liver cells,

. . . and allow excessive insulin into the circulation,

. . . which retains salt and plumps up the blood volume,

. . . that causes the blood pressure to rise so high that it

. . . bursts the wall of an artery in the brain causing a deep STROKE.

CHAPTER 14

WHAT'S EATING YOU . . . CRAVINGS & FOOD SENSITIVITIES

Summary

Here we look at appetite, our natural cravings for salty and sweet, and how they must be managed. Then there are those modern phenomena, food allergies and food sensitivities . . . which we will consider, too.

Hunger is a natural drive directing us to look for something to eat. Few people develop weight problems on food that is dull or bland, and laboratory rats do not get fat on biscuits of chow. When tasty human food is substituted, however, the rats get fat. Making food products irresistible to these natural inclinations of sweet and salty is an important objective of food processors, ever alert for flavorful additives. Weight-prone individuals must become wary of the flavor trap.

Mother Nature has hardwired us to crave *sweet things* (they are ripe and comfortable to digest) *salty things* (ancestral forms from a salty sea adapted to a salt-scarce land), *creamy* (calorie-rich seed oil in a calorie-scarce world) and *crunchy* (jaws and teeth need workouts). Common foods that are craved and lead to binge eating are typically sweet or salty or crunchy. Sugar is blamed, and most long-term weight control successes in my practice did not allow themselves to eat anything sweet, nor keep anything sweet handy. They know it would awaken the beast within. Substitutes were found and new habits learned such as a granola bar or piece of fruit as a better response to the old sugar trigger.

There is also mounting evidence that today's 24/7 work and recreation life sets us up for binge eating and obesity. We are daytime creatures with hundreds of clocks in the tissues of our bodies that keep all our metabolic functions synchronized to daylight. Sunlight triggers receptors in the eyes, and connections to the brain keep tissue clocks in synchrony. Experimental animals fed on the 'sleep sides' of their sleep/wake cycles develop bubble bellies on the same food intake that maintained them lean and well when eaten during the 'waking side.' Like other mammals, we function best during daylight hours. Eyes that are stimulated by daylight, signal the brain's timekeepers to harmonize our clocks, directing us to look for breakfast in the morning and a place to sleep when the light fails.

Twenty healthy young adults volunteered for a most enlightening 'sleep/wake' study. For three weeks, they slept only 6 hours of every 24-hour cycle. In a controlled environment of constant dim light, they cycled through 28-hour days on 6 hours of sleep. They grew irritable. Their blood sugars began to rise, their metabolic rates fell, and they gained weight. Some had food cravings. Projected out over a year from the brief test period, the weight gain added up to 10 pounds each.

Once the study was complete, they remained under observation but now slept for 10 hours on a normal 24 hour day/night cycle. Dispositions improved and blood sugars fell. The take-away mesage: sleep deprivation is probably common in binge eaters. Confine your eating and drinking to the daylight hours.

SOME SIMPLE CRAVINGS-CRUSHERS

A few alternatives to the tub of ice cream or box of cookies
Allow 30 minutes for some degree of satisfaction to develop, and if it does not, repeat.

A SPOONFUL OF PEANUT BUTTER

MICROWAVED YAM SPOONED UP WITH NONFAT MAYO

EGG-WHITE OMELETTE WITH MUSHROOMS OR GREEN PEAS

FIST-SIZED BOWL OF BERRIES CREAMED WITH PROTEIN SHAKE

FIST OF MICROWAVED GREEN BEANS AND SLIVERED ALMONDS

SMALL CAN OF TUNA/CHICKEN MASHED WITH NONFAT MAYO,

MICROWAVED BRUSSELS SPROUTS WITH DIJON MUSTARD

HOT BOWL OF RICE WITH SOY SAUCE

MICROWAVED POTATO & ONION: CHUNKED, NONFAT MAYO

DEVELOP YOUR OWN CRAVINGS CRUSHER

Cravings for sweet or salty foods are not addictions in the pharmacological sense, but built-in preferences from a dim and distant past. They had survival value, and will not go away. It is best to never take "just one bite" of any such food again.

Although we tend to think drugs when considering addiction, a degree of chemical dependence can develop on food items like coffee, colas and chocolate. Probably one person in three has addictive tendencies (including to gambling, even jogging and shopping). Any disturbed peace of mind can set the stage for a needed fix, but the need most often is for something to lift the spirits and restore energy.

Weight-prone individuals are inclined to eat when feeling tired or depressed. Chemical energies in the brain are down, and the emotional battery too low to resist the urge always drumming within. Naturally lean individuals do not experience this constant low-grade hunger signal, indeed, they must often remind themselves to eat, tending to miss meals otherwise. When depressed or tired they can remain indifferent to food. Exhaustion and fatigue seems to kill any inclination to eat. They are different from weight-prone individuals who turn to food for emotional energy when down or tired.

For permanent weight control, sugary and sweet things should no longer, ever be at hand – no cookies, candy, ice cream etc. ever again. Diet sodas too, are best avoided as they keep the sweet tooth sharp. Natural, inborn signals cannot be removed, only modified by conditioned habit change, which is do-able. Human breast milk is sweet. Experimentally, when less-sweet breast milk is substituted the baby rejects it at first, but within two weeks of a substitution, the baby prefers it over naturally sweet.

Digestion is a process of controlled food flow along some 25 feet of intestinal tubing. It is divided into three organ-stages: the *stomach*, the *small bowel* or intestine and the large bowel or *colon*. In the stomach, food that has been chewed and mixed with saliva and swallowed, enters a stomach that produces acid digesting enzymes. Food spends perhaps an hour there, becoming liquefied before being squirted on into the small bowel. More digestive enzymes and chemicals are added from the liver and pancreas, to work on stomach output over the next 12 hours. During this passage along some 20 feet of small bowel, nutrients become released from food and absorbed into the body. Juices from the wall of the small intestine thoroughly liquefy everything they can before delivering the residue mush into the colon. Digestion has taken place, water and minerals are now re-absorbed. Indigestible food residue is food fiber.

The normal digestive tract teems with bacteria and viruses picked up from the environment. Indeed, there are more bacteria inhabiting the bowel than there are cells in the human body. They react with us (their host) and help maintain our health. New research is teasing out previously unrecognized ways they contribute to a strong immune system and a normal gut. It is an area of intense scientific interest that holds promise for an even better understanding of the toxic waist.

Research teams around the world are pondering the microbes in this tunnel, and one team leader is Chinese. He works in Shanghai. After a decade of training in the U.S., he developed a bubble belly, and an increase in his blood pressure and cholesterol. He began to monitor the population of microbes in his own digestive tract, discovering that they had become "American" during his time here. He returned to his native diet and restored them to a "Chinese" pattern within six weeks. By changing his diet to fruits, vegetables and whole grain foods, he converted the microbial population in his gut. Without restricting calories, he eliminated his toxic waist, his elevated blood pressure and cholesterol on a diet that involved whole grains, kale, yams, seaweed and bitter melon. To colleagues in America, his e-mail signatures now end: *Eat right, keep fit, live long, die quick.*

NEXT UP:
FOOD AS A SOURCE OF ILL-HEALTH BEYOND GLUTEN SENSITIVITY

Food allergies and food sensitivities are different clinical problems. Food allergies can be life-threatening. They often provoke acute abdominal discomfort, skin hives or wheezing. Their reactions are dramatic and tightly tied to food exposure. A relationship is quickly recognized that requires specialist medical attention. The allergy can often be confirmed by a series of skin tests.

Food sensitivity is different. It is rarely life-threatening and usually shows nothing on skin testing. Symptoms include: nasal stuffiness, low-grade headaches, skin itching, abdominal tenderness and bloating, water-weight gain. Other individuals crave foods to which they have become sensitive, typically wheat and dairy products. Eating them can provoke binge eating. In this type of food intolerance, the symptoms are not immediate and less obvious, developing a day or two after the food is eaten, and may consist only of fatigue and depression. Binge eating the offending food is common, and sensitivities may contribute to a weight problem in susceptible people.

Identifying food sensitivity depends on the history, and a dietary challenge. All your usual foods must be withdrawn, then taken in challenge after two weeks on the Exclusion Food Diet outlined below and on the next page.

THE EXCLUSION DIET FOR FOOD SENSITIVITY

BEVERAGES: water, tea, grape juice and pineapple juice no sugar added

CEREALS: oatmeal or rice without milk and served with any of the above drinks

BREADS: Rye Crisp plain, barley plain, rye or potato flour bread

FRUITS: grapes, apricots, plums, cherries, apples, pineapples

MEATS: lamb or well done beef - gray, not pink

VEGETABLES: carrots, beets, celery, yams, lettuce, potatoes, broccoli, beets, olives

SEASONINGS: salt, ginger, vanilla extract, cinnamon - avoid other herbs and spicess

WEETENERS: Nutrasweet or honeyIf you suspect you have a food sensitivity and want to determine what foods might be causing your problems, eat only from the selection outlined above for 2 weeks, no mixtures of foods, no alcohol and no aspirin. For aches or pains use Tylenol. Feeling poorly over the first few days is a good sign. Your system is clearing itself of old toxic products. By the second week you should feel as though a storm has passed and you're in the clear. Once you feel clear, eat some of the suspect food as a test and see.

A patient of mine had been trying to lose the same 15 pounds all her adult life. Now they're gone and through the simplest of expedients: she avoids wheat and wheat flour in her diet. She is a lawyer with a jaundiced view of human nature and skeptical of the whole concept of food sensitivity. At first she denied any symptoms but on close questioning admitted to episodes of sneezing during tree pollen time and a swollen face and tight rings whenever she drank certain wines. She could gain as much as 8 pounds from a single serving of certain foods, and agreed to go on the elimination diet, discovering that she reacted badly to wheat products, whether in bread or breakfast cereal or cake flour. The reaction had kept her almost permanently puffed with 15 pounds of fluid.

Follow your nose would be a reasonable guide to any effect of food on the digestive tract. We seldom think of the nose as the leading edge of our digestive tracts, but it recognizes aromatic food and starts digestive juices flowing. Like the gut, the nose can become inflamed and swollen when exposed to sensitizing foods. Skeptics call the reaction "nasal stuffiness," dismiss it as a virus cold, or flu, or the "old sinus" acting up. Sometimes they are right. It might be the stuffiness of a virus or a cold or flu. Often, however, it is the congestive response of an injured digestive tract, injured by apparently innocent food ingredients such as milk products, wheat, corn, coffee or citrus fruits.

BE WARY OF ANY FOOD YOU FEEL STRONGLY ABOUT

Notes...

CHAPTER 15

FINALLY, TIME FOR A LITTLE

GOOD

CLEAN

FUN . . .

One-Dish Meals

Vegetables

Broccoli Bake

2 cups steamed broccoli
1/3 cup dry curd cottage cheese
1 tsp lemon juice
1 tsp grated onion
Parmesan Crumb Mix
Combine cottage cheese, lemon juice and grated onion in the blender.
Blend well. Spread over broccoli. Sprinkle with Parmesan-crumb mix.
Broil until golden. Each serving equals one cup.

Broiled Tomatoes

Sprinkle sliced tomatoes with Parmesan-Crumbs and an herb seasoning
blend. Broil until crumb mix is lightly toasted. Three med. tomatoes
equal a fist serving.

Dilled New Potatoes

Scrub tiny new potatoes (leave skins on, if desired).
Simmer gently in Chicken Stock until they're done.
Sprinkle with dill, dried or fresh.

Carrots & Scallions

2-2 1/2 cups steamed carrots, sliced or juilenned
1 tsp Ginger-Garlic Oil

2-3 chopped scallions (green part only)
Briefly saute scallions in oil. Add the carrots and heat through.

Green Beans With Almonds

1 pound trenched green beans (may be frozen)
Chicken Stock*
1 tsp Ginger-Garlic Oil
1/2 cup toasted almonds
(sliced or slivered)
Cook green beans in chicken stock until barely tender. Drain. Toss with oil, add almonds and toss again.

Stuffed Mushrooms

1 lb. large mushrooms
2 T coarsely ground
blanched almonds
1 garlic clove, pressed
t tsp dried tarragon
2 slices whole wheat bread
made into bread crumbs
2 T plain low-fat yogurt
Remove stems from mushrooms. Saute caps lightly. Cool. Combine remaining ingredients and stuff into caps. Sprinkle 1 T Parmesan over caps and broil.

Carrots & Brussel Sprouts

2 cups steamed carrots, sliced
1 cup brussels sprouts
1/2 cup Chicken Stock
pinch sugar-if necessary

lemon juice to taste
pepper to taste

Bring chicken stock to boil. Add brussel sprouts (and sugar) and simmer until done. Drain. Add carrots and lemon juice; heat through. Season to taste. Each serving equals one cup.

Ratatouille

4 zucchini, sliced
1-11/2 lb. egg plant, unpeeled & sliced
2 cups canned tomatoes, plus liquid
2 T parsley, fresh & chopped
2 tsp basil, dried 1-2 T olive oil
2 medium onions, sliced
2 cloves garlic, crushed
2 green peppers, sliced
1 cup chopped celery
ground pepper to taste

In a heavy pot, saute in oil: garlic, onion, green pepper, celery until limp. Add everything else, cover and cook over low heat until soft. Remove lid, cook until liquid is reduced. Serve hot, lukewarm or cold.

Pineapple-Stuffed Squash

1 8-ounce can crushed pineapple 2 small acorn squash (about 1 pound)
in own juice, drained. ground cinnamon. Or fresh pineapple cut into small pieces

Cut each squash in half lengthwise and remove seeds. Spoon pineapple into squash cavities. In a 10" skillet over medium heat, in 1/2" of water, place squash, cut-side up. Heat to boiling then cover and reduce heat to low. Simmer 20 minutes or until tender. To serve, sprinkle cinnamon over pineapple. One half a squash equals a one fist serving.

Potato-Onion Bake

2-3 potatoes unpeeled, but scrubbed and thinly sliced
1-2 medium onions, thinly sliced
1/2-1 cup Chicken Stock*
1/4 **cup Parmesan-Crumb Mixture***

Arrange the potatoes and onions in a shallow baking dish. Barely cover with chicken stock. Sprinkle with Parmesan-Crumb mix and bake uncovered at 375 degrees for 45-60 minutes, or until tender.

Sherried Sweet Potatoes

3 sweet potatoes
1 T Sherry
1/2 cup orange juice
1 T brown sugar, if necessary orange zest and nutmeg to taste

Bake sweet potatoes in skins, at 375 degrees for 45-60 minues, or until soft to touch. Cool and peel. Mash with remaining ingredients until smooth.

A Breakfast Sweet Potato

Microwave one yam fist-sized 10-12 minutes. Let stand. Cut in half. Spoon up with tips of chilled mayo (non-fat).

Soups

Chicken Stock

2 lbs chicken bones, wings & backs or a 3 lb fryer
2 large onions, Including skins
1-2 bay leaves
3-4 peppercorns1/4 bunch fresh parsley
1/2 bunch fresh dill

Clean and rinse chicken, discarding skin and loose fat. Cover with water in a pot; bring to boil for 2 minutes. Discard liquid and add fresh water and remaining ingredients; bring to boil, lower heat and simmer for 3-4 hours. Pour stock into container, cool to room temperature and refrigerate overnight. Remove fat; strain stock through cheesecloth or fine mesh. Freeze strained stock in ice cube trays. Store in plastic bags; 6 cubes equal 1 cup.

Split Pea/Bean/Lentil Soup

1 quart Chicken Stock*
1 cup dried lentils, beans or split peas
1 carrot, chopped
2 ribs of celery, chopped
1 small potato, diced
1/2 green pepper, chopped
1-2 garlic cloves, mashed
1 T dried basil 1 bay leaf
ground pepper to taste
balsamic vinegar, or vinegar of your choice
(Optional: 1 cup chopped spinach or cabbage)

Bring all ingredients to boil, cover and simmer for 11/2 hours.

Tomato and Barley Soup

1 quart Chicken Stock
1/2 cup medium barley
1-2 ribs celery, chopped
1/4 cup chopped onion
1-2 cups chopped tomato or
1 lb. canned tomatoes plus liquid
Bring to boil, cover and simmer 60-90 minutes. Each serving equals one cup

Minestrone

1 tap oil
1/2 cup chopped onion
1 clove garlic, mashed
1 carrot, sliced
1 rib celery, sliced
1 cup chopped cabbage
1 cup tomatoes, chopped with liquid
1/2 zucchini sliced
1/2 tsp sugar, basil, oregano, pepper to taste
1 cup beans (kidney, pinto, white) cooked and drained
1/2 cup uncooked curly noodles
3 cups Chicken Stock*
Saute onion and garlic in oil. Add stock, vegetables, seasonings and bring to a boil, simmer 10 minutes. Add noodles and cook until noodles are done, about 10-15 minutes.

Turkey Chili

1 lb. ground turkey
chili powder to taste

1 cup Chili Salsa*
1 med. onion, chopped
2 cups cooked kidney beans
1 can stewed tomatoes

Brown ground turkey with onion. Add stewed tomatoes, chili salsa, and chili powder. Cover and simmer for 60 min. Add beans and cook for 30 minutes longer.

Gazpacho

1 clove garlic, peeled
1 medium onion, quartered
1 cucumber, peeled and cut up
3-4 tomatoes (may use canned)
1 green pepper, seeded and cut into 4 pieces

Combine in a food processor everything but the liquid ingredients; blend. Add liquids. Serve well-chilled with croutons.

Broccoli Cheese & Potato

1 C broccoli flowerets, steamed
1 fist-sized microwaved potato, peeled and chunked
2 T 1% cottage cheese
Parmesan Cheese, Ground pepper

Spinach Pie

2 cloves garlic, mashed
2 cups chopped onion
1/2 cup Chicken Stock
2 cups sliced mushrooms
1 whole egg 1 egg white

Cook garlic and onions in chicken stock until tender. Add mushrooms and reduce liquid to 1 T. Cool. Blend with eggs for 15 seconds. Combine mushroom mixture, spinach, crumb mix, and seasonings. Pour into a lightly greased 8" or 9" pie pan and bake for 45 minutes at 325 degrees. Each serving equals one-eighth of the pie.

Simple Stir-Fries

Starting the night before or that morning, have 2-3 cups of vegetables (any three or more) cleaned and trimmed to size, preferably thinly sliced. Suggested vegetables (fresh or frozen) include:

carrots celery green pepper scallions cauliflower snow pea pods broccoli mushrooms bok choy cabbage zucchini brussels sprouts or any other of your choice

At cooking time, heat 1-2 tsp of Ginger-Garlic Oil* and 2-3 T Chicken Stock and 1-2 T sherry or sake in a wok or skillet. Use the highest setting. Add the vegetables and toss and stir until tender/crisp— don't over-cook. Remove with a slotted spoon. To the liquid in the pan, add: 1 T cornstarch dissolved in 1/3 cup cool water or chicken stock. Cook over low heat, stirring until slightly thickened. Sparingly add tamari to taste. Return vegetables to the skillet and heat through. Serve over your choice of grain or beans . . .especially good over barley, bulgur or rice.

Kaluha Chicken

1 whole large chicken breast (skinned and boned)
1 large bunch broccoli, cut up
2-3 large carrots, sliced
1 cup or more Chicken Stock
3 tsp. cornstarch
2 large cloves garlic, crushed
1 tsp. grated ginger root

1/2 cup Kaluha or any coffee liqueur 2 T soy sauce
Cut chicken into 1-inch pieces. Combine soy sauce, 1/2 cup Kaluha, 1 clove garlic, and 1/2 tsp. ginger. Add to the chicken and marinate for few hours. Meanwhile, steam carrots and broccoli in a microwave for 3 min. Heat stock, 1 clove garlic, and V2 tsp. ginger in a wok. Add chicken and cook until done. Add vegetables and cook a few minutes more. Add cornstarch and Kaluha to the stock, then add to the wok. Stir until bubbly. Each serving includes 1/2 chicken breast.

Chicken Cacciatore

2 chicken breasts, skinned
2 cups stewed tomatoes
1-2 cloves garlic, mashed
1 cup chopped onion
1/2 cup whole wheat flour
1/2-1 tsp dried basil
1/2 tsp thyme
1/2 cup dry red wine
Place chicken breasts and flour in broil-in-bag and shake. Discardexcess flour. Close bag with a twister, and cut three V2" slits inbag. Bake at 425 degrees for 10-15 minutes or until lightly brown-ed. Remove chicken, place in a baking dish, and pour the sauceover it. Cover and bake for one hour or more at 375 degrees.
Sauce: cook onion and garlic in the juice from the tomatoes untiltender. Add everything else, bring to a boil and simmer gently for5 minutes. Each serving equals V2 chicken breast.

Spinach Lasagne

Prepare: 12 whole wheat lasagne noodles, cooked
Combine:

10 oz. frozen spinach, thawed 1 CUP low-fat cottage cheese (1%) and chopped 2 T parmesan cheese
OR: 1 pound fresh spinach, grind of pepper steamed and pressed dry V4 tsP nutmeg

Spread the noodles with spinach filling and roll up and lay in a casserole. Blend together sauce ingredients (below)and pour over spinach rolls.

1/2 pound mushrooms, sliced 3 cups tomato sauce
1 tsp basil 1 cup chopped onion
1 tsp oregano 2 cloves garlic, crushed
1/2 **tsp rosemary**
Cover and bake at 350 degrees for one hour

Baked Filet of Fish, Vegetables

Filet of Sole etc. pepper, tarragon, basil, or thyme
number of servings-4 oz. each and some paprika
light white wine 1 cup vegetables of your choice
lemon juice per fish filet

Place fish in a baking dish. Sprinkle with spices of your choiceas listed above. Pour lemon juice and wine over fish. Place chop-ped vegetables, such as broccoli, carrots, cauliflower, green pep-per, onion and mushrooms, around the fish. Bake at 350 degreesuntil vegetables are done and the fish is flaky.

Tuna & Green Beans

1 oz. tuna, fist of green beans, steamed
1 sm. tomato, chopped
Ground pepper Parmesan cheese

Pesto Pasta Sauce

1 pkg Butter Buds, diluted
2 cloves garlic to taste
3-4 T sunflower seeds
1/2 **tsp pepper**
2 cups fresh basil
1/2 **cup Parmesan Cheese**

In a covered blender, process Butter Buds and garlic on high speed until smooth. Remove inner cap or cover of blender and gradually add seeds and pepper. Blend until smooth. A little at a time, add basil. Stir mixture down with a scraper and add Parmesan Cheese.

Chicken L'Orange Amandine

1-2 whole chicken breasts, boned halved and skinned
1/4 cup whole wheat flour
1/2t **tsp paprika**
1 tsp grated orange peel
1 T vegetable oil
1 clove garlic, mashed

Pound chicken breasts between waxed paper sheets until thin.

Combine flour, paprika and orange peel in paper bag, and addchicken. Shake to coat. Brown the breasts in oil in a skillet.

Transfer to a shallow baking dish. Add garlic to the skillet and cook, stirring for a minute. Add wine, orange juice, thyme and pepper and heat.

Pour this over the chicken and bake at 350 degrees for15 minutes. Add orange slices and bake 15 minutes more. Sprinkle almonds over chicken.

Moussaka

1 large egg plant, sliced half-inch thick
1 large onion, finely chopped
2 cloves garlic, mashed
1 1/2 cups cooked brown rice
1 cup cooked soy beans, pureed
3 T tomato paste
1/2 cup red wine
1/2 **cup chopped fresh parsley**
1/2 **cup each basil and rosemary**
tsp cinnamon freshly ground pepper

Bake eggplant slices until soft at 350 degrees. Meanwhile saute onion and garlic in 1 T vegetable stock until onion is soft. Add beans, rice, herbs, pepper, tomato paste and wine. Mix well. Put a thin layer of bean-rice mixture in bottom of a casserole, add eggplant slices, then the rest of the bean-rice mixture. In a sauce pan, melt the margarine and stir in the flour. Whisk smooth. Add milk slowly, and keep stirring until mixture becomes thick. Remove from heat and stir in the cottage cheese and nutmeg. Add eggs and mix well. Pour this over the casserole layers. Top with breadcrumbs and Parmesan and bake in a 375 degree oven for 40-60 minutes, or until golden. Cool a little before serving. Each serving equals one cup.

www.ingramcontent.com/pod-product-compliance
Lightning Source LLC
Chambersburg PA
CBHW072310290526
45794CB00002B/597